Topics in Obstetrics and Gynecology Ultrasound

Guest Editor

PHYLLIS GLANC, MD

ULTRASOUND CLINICS

www.ultrasound.theclinics.com

Consulting Editor
VIKRAM S. DOGRA, MD

January 2012 • Volume 7 • Number 1

SAUNDERS an imprint of ELSEVIER, Inc.

W.B. SAUNDERS COMPANY
A Division of Elsevier Inc.

1600 John F. Kennedy Boulevard ● Suite 1800 ● Philadelphia, Pennsylvania 19103-2899

http://www.theclinics.com

ULTRASOUND CLINICS Volume 7, Number 1
January 2012 ISSN 1556-858X, ISBN-13: 978-1-4557-3945-5

Editor: Donald Mumford

Ultrasound Clinics (ISSN 1556-858X) is published quarterly by W.B. Saunders, 360 Park Avenue South, New York, NY 10010-1710. Months of publication are January, April, July, and October. Business and editorial offices: 1600 John F. Kennedy Boulevard, Suite 1800, Philadelphia, Pennsylvania 19103-2899. Accounting and circulation offices: 6277 Sea Harbor Drive, Orlando, FL 32887-4800. Periodicals postage paid at New York, NY, and additional mailing offices. Subscription prices are $243 per year for (US individuals), $297 per year for (US institutions), $139 per year for (US students and residents), $273 per year for (Canadian individuals), $332 per year for (Canadian institutions), $291 per year for (international individuals), $332 per year for (international institutions), and $139 per year for (Canadian and foreign students/residents). To receive student/resident rate, orders must be accompanied by name of affiliated institution, date of term, and the signature of program/residency coordinator on institution letterhead. Orders will be billed at individual rate until proof of status is received. Foreign air speed delivery is included in all Clinics subscription prices. All prices are subject to change without notice. **POSTMASTER:** Send address changes to *Ultrasound Clinics,* Elsevier Health Sciences Division, Subscription Customer Service, 3251 Riverport Lane, Maryland Heights, MO 63043. **Customer Service (orders, claims, online, change of address): Telephone: 1-800-654-2452 (U.S. and Canada); 314-447-8871 (outside U.S. and Canada). Fax: 314-447-8029. E-mail: journalscustomerservice-usa@elsevier.com (for print support); journalsonlinesupport-usa@elsevier.com (for online support).**

Reprints: For copies of 100 or more, of articles in this publication, please contact the Commercial Reprints Department, Elsevier Inc., 360 Park Avenue South, New York, NY 10010-1710. Tel.: (+1) 212-633-3812; Fax: (+1) 212-462-1935; E-mail: reprints@elsevier.com.

Printed and bound by CPI Group (UK) Ltd, Croydon, CR0 4YY
Transferred to Digital Print 2012

Contributors

CONSULTING EDITOR

VIKRAM S. DOGRA, MD
Professor of Radiology, Urology, and
Biomedical Engineering, Director of Ultrasound
and Associate Chair for Education and
Research, Department of Imaging Sciences,
University of Rochester School of Medicine
and Dentistry, Rochester, New York

GUEST EDITOR

PHYLLIS GLANC, MD, FRCPC (C)
Associate Professor, Abdominal Imaging
Division, Department of Medical Imaging;
Department of Obstetrics & Gynecology,
University of Toronto; Co-Director, Obstetrical
Ultrasound Centre, Sunnybrook Health
Science Centre, Toronto, Ontario, Canada

AUTHORS

REUVEN ACHIRON, MD
Department of Obstetrics and Gynecology,
The Chaim Sheba Medical Center,
Tel-Hashomer, Ramat Gan; Affiliated
with the Sackler Faculty of Medicine,
Tel Aviv University, Israel

ROCHELLE F. ANDREOTTI, MD
Clinical Professor of Radiology, Associate
Clinical Professor of Obstetrics and
Gynecology, Department of Obstetrics
and Gynecology; Department of Radiology
and Radiological Sciences, Vanderbilt
University Medical Center, Nashville,
Tennessee

CARRIE B. BETEL, MD
Assistant Professor, Department of Medical
Imaging, University of Toronto, Sunnybrook
Health Sciences Centre, Toronto, Ontario,
Canada

BRIAN D. COLEY, MD
Radiologist-in-Chief, Professor of Radiology,
Cincinnati Children's Hospital Medical Center,
Cincinnati, Ohio

MANJIRI K. DIGHE, MD
Associate Professor of Radiology,
Chief in Body Imaging and Director
of Ultrasound, University of Washington,
Seattle, Washington

THEODORE J. DUBINSKY, MD
Laurence A. Mack Endowed Professor
of Radiology, Department of Radiology,
University of Washington, Seattle,
Washington

ARTHUR C. FLEISCHER, MD
Professor of Radiology, Department
of Radiology and Radiological Sciences;
Professor of Obstetrics and Gynecology,
Department of Obstetrics and Gynecology,
Vanderbilt University Medical Center,
Nashville, Tennessee

MARY C. FRATES, MD
Associate Professor of Radiology, Department of Radiology, Harvard Medical School; Assistant Director of Ultrasound, Brigham and Women's Hospital, Boston, Massachusetts

LIAT GINDES, MD
Department of Obstetrics and Gynecology, The Chaim Sheba Medical Center, Tel-Hashomer, Ramat Gan; Affiliated with the Sackler Faculty of Medicine, Tel Aviv University, Israel

PHYLLIS GLANC, MD, FRCPC (C)
Associate Professor, Department of Medical Imaging, Abdominal Imaging Division; Department of Obstetrics & Gynecology, University of Toronto; Co-Director, Obstetrical Ultrasound Centre, Sunnybrook Health Science Centre, Toronto, Ontario, Canada

ERIC JAUNIAUX, MD, PhD, FRCOG
Academic Department of Obstetrics and Gynaecology, Institute for Women Health at University College London, London, United Kingdom

DAVOR JURKOVIC, MD, FRCOG
Academic Department of Obstetrics & Gynaecology, UCL Institute for Women's Health, University College London, London, United Kingdom

JEAN H. LEE, MD
Assistant Professor of Radiology, University of Washington, Seattle, Washington

ANDREJ LYSHCHIK, MD, PhD
Fellow, Interventional Radiology, Department of Radiology and Radiological Sciences, Vanderbilt University Medical Center, Nashville, Tennessee

CAITLIN T. MCGREGOR, MD, FRCP
Assistant Professor, Division of Abdominal Imaging, Department of Medical Imaging, Sunnybrook Health Sciences Centre, University of Toronto, Toronto, Ontario, Canada

ORI NEVO, MD
Assistant Professor, Division of Maternal Fetal Medicine; Co-Director Department of Obstetrics and Gynecology, Obstetrical Ultrasound Centre, Sunnybrook Health Sciences Centre, University of Toronto, Toronto, Ontario, Canada

MARIA PIRANER, MD
Fellow, Women's Imaging, Department of Radiology and Radiological Sciences, Vanderbilt University Medical Center, Nashville, Tennessee

DOLORES H. PRETORIUS, MD
Department of Radiology, University of California, San Diego; Thornton Hospital, La Jolla, California

N.J. SEBIRE, MD, MRCPath
Trophoblastic Disease Unit, Department of Cancer Medicine, Charing Cross Hospital, London, United Kingdom

MICHELLE SWER, BSc, MBBS, MRCOG
Academic Department of Obstetrics & Gynaecology, UCL Institute for Women's Health, University College London, London, United Kingdom

ALINA WEISSMANN-BRENNER, MD
Department of Obstetrics and Gynecology, The Chaim Sheba Medical Center, Tel-Hashomer, Ramat Gan; Affiliated with the Sackler Faculty of Medicine, Tel Aviv University, Israel

Contents

The prenatal diagnosis of congenital heart disease is of great importance, due to its high incidence at birth and elevated rates of neonatal mortality. Demonstration of the 4-chamber, 3-vessel and trachea, and sagittal aortic arch views is necessary for complete fetal cardiac assessment. Abnormal number, arrangement, size, and alignment of the blood vessels are indicators of anomalies. The objective of this article is to assess the added value of the 3-vessel and trachea views along with the cardiac arches in conjunction with the 4-chamber view in fetal echocardiography. Careful sonographic cardiac evaluation may improve prenatal diagnosis of congenital heart disease.

When performing obstetric ultrasonography, errors can occur. This article reviews the common mistakes made in measurements and survey images.

Ultrasound plays a central role in the modern management of early pregnancy complications, and is important in the identification, diagnosis, and surveillance of gestational trophoblastic disease (GTD). The term GTD is confusing, encompassing the range of entities in this group, such as complete hydatidiform mole, partial hydatidiform mole, invasive mole, malignant choriocarcinoma, and placental site trophoblastic tumor. The role of ultrasound in their management varies according to the specific entity, but, for the clinician, the most common and important aspect is the use of ultrasound examination for the identification of pregnancies complicated by hydatidiform mole.

Threatened miscarriage (TM) is associated with an increased risk of adverse obstetric and perinatal outcomes. Ultrasound enables a conclusive diagnosis in most normal pregnancies and early pregnancy abnormalities. Maternal serum biochemistry can help to predict early pregnancy outcomes. Ultrasound findings and maternal serum biochemistry, together with the clinical history, provide valuable information about the prognosis of TM and are important to determine potential management options. More studies on these common early pregnancy complications should enable better management protocols and new therapeutic guidelines to improve the perinatal outcome in women at higher risk of abnormal pregnancy outcome.

The human fetus reaches major developmental milestones during the first trimester of pregnancy, and most of the known birth defects appear during this time. Late first-trimester ultrasound allows us to achieve a high detection rate of congenital malformations when performed transvaginally by experienced operators. Although late first-trimester transvaginal anatomy has not been introduced as a routine examination in most countries, the authors recommend the procedure to women at risk for fetal anomalies and think it may also be beneficial to obese gravid women. Further development of 3-dimensional ultrasound technologies may be efficacious in future first-trimester anatomy scans.

This article reviews cystic ovarian lesions, with a focus on sonographic characteristics. Ultrasonographic techniques and approaches are described, with reference to other imaging modalities. More detailed features of specific diagnoses are presented, and, specifically, tumors of low malignant potential are discussed in more detail. Clinical considerations and management are also discussed.

Recent improvements in sonographic techniques such as color Doppler sonography and volumetric or three-dimensional sonography provide improved depiction of ovarian and uterine vascularity. This article discusses and illustrates the clinical applications of these new techniques for evaluating ovarian masses, detection of adnexal torsion, uterine fibroids, polyps, and certain vascular abnormalities. Potential uses of contrast-enhanced transvaginal sonography are also addressed.

As in adults, ultrasound is the first and often most definitive imaging modality for the evaluation of the female pelvis. Common reasons for clinical referral include evaluation of pelvic pain or a pelvic mass, abnormalities of puberty, and disorders of sexual development. An understanding of the basics of gynecologic embryology is necessary to understand congenital malformations that often predispose to these clinical scenarios.

Uterine bleeding in postmenopausal women is caused by endometrial atrophy, endometrial hyperplasia, endometrial polyp, submucosal leiomyoma, and endometrial cancer. Although most postmenopausal uterine bleeding is attributed to benign causes, the most common presenting symptom of endometrial cancer is uterine bleeding. Endovaginal sonography is generally accepted as an initial diagnostic tool to evaluate endometrium. It allows triaging patients who need endometrial biopsy and histologic diagnosis versus hysterosonography and hysteroscopy. Hysterosonography can be useful not only in the confirmation and characterization of focal endometrial pathologic conditions but it can also provide guidance to localize and treat focal endometrial pathologic conditions.

Ultrasound of the bowel requires significant expertise but is useful in premenopausal women presenting to an ultrasound department with pelvic pain. Gynecologic and gastrointestinal causes of pelvic pain can cause similar clinical presentations. This article includes a review of the anatomy of the gastrointestinal tract and bowel wall in addition to the techniques used to perform a thorough evaluation of the bowel with ultrasound. Gastrointestinal causes of pelvic pain are discussed, including appendicitis, diverticulitis, inflammatory bowel disease, epiploic appendagitis, omental infarction, and infection.

Ultrasound Clinics

THE CLINICS ARE NOW AVAILABLE ONLINE!

Access your subscription at:
www.theclinics.com

GOAL STATEMENT

The goal of the *Ultrasound Clinics* is to keep practicing radiologists and radiology residents up to date with current clinical practice in ultrasound by providing timely articles reviewing the state of the art in patient care.

ACCREDITATION

The *Ultrasound Clinics* is planned and implemented in accordance with the Essential Areas and Policies of the Accreditation Council for Continuing Medical Education (ACCME) through the joint sponsorship of the University of Virginia School of Medicine and Elsevier. The University of Virginia School of Medicine is accredited by the ACCME to provide continuing medical education for physicians.

The University of Virginia School of Medicine designates this enduring material activity for a maximum of 15 *AMA PRA Category 1 Credit*(s)™ for each issue, 60 credits per year. Physicians should claim only the credit commensurate with the extent of their participation in the activity.

The American Medical Association has determined that physicians not licensed in the US who participate in this CME enduring material activity are eligible for a maximum of 15 *AMA PRA Category 1 Credit*(s)™ for each issue, 60 credits per year.

Credit can be earned by reading the text material, taking the CME examination online at http://www.theclinics.com/home/cme, and completing the evaluation. After taking the test, you will be required to review any and all incorrect answers. Following completion of the test and evaluation, your credit will be awarded and you may print your certificate.

FACULTY DISCLOSURE/CONFLICT OF INTEREST

The University of Virginia School of Medicine, as an ACCME accredited provider, endorses and strives to comply with the Accreditation Council for Continuing Medical Education (ACCME) Standards of Commercial Support, Commonwealth of Virginia statutes, University of Virginia policies and procedures, and associated federal and private regulations and guidelines on the need for disclosure and monitoring of proprietary and financial interests that may affect the scientific integrity and balance of content delivered in continuing medical education activities under our auspices.

The University of Virginia School of Medicine requires that all CME activities accredited through this institution be developed independently and be scientifically rigorous, balanced and objective in the presentation/discussion of its content, theories and practices.

All authors/editors participating in an accredited CME activity are expected to disclose to the readers relevant financial relationships with commercial entities occurring within the past 12 months (such as grants or research support, employee, consultant, stock holder, member of speakers bureau, etc.). The University of Virginia School of Medicine will employ appropriate mechanisms to resolve potential conflicts of interest to maintain the standards of fair and balanced education to the reader. Questions about specific strategies can be directed to the Office of Continuing Medical Education, University of Virginia School of Medicine, Charlottesville, Virginia.

The faculty and staff of the University of Virginia Office of Continuing Medical Education have no financial affiliations to disclose.

The authors/editors listed below have identified no professional or financial affiliations for themselves or their spouse/partner:

Reuven Achiron, MD; Rochelle F. Andreotti, MD; Carrie B. Betel, MD; Brian D. Coley, MD; Manjiri K. Dighe, MD; Theodore J. Dubinsky, MD; Arthur C. Fleischer, MD; Mary C. Frates, MD; Liat Gindes, MD; Phyllis Glanc, MD, FRCPC (C) (Guest Editor); Eric Jauniaux, MD, PhD, FRCOG; Davor Jurkovic, MD, FRCOG; Jean H. Lee, MD; Caitlin T. McGregor, MD, FRCP; Donald Mumford, (Acquisitions Editor); Ori Nevo, MD; Maria Piraner, MD; N.J. Sebire, MD, MRCPath; Michelle Swer, BSc, MBBS, MRCOG; and Alina Weissmann-Brenner, MD.

The authors/editors listed below have identified the following professional or financial affiliations for themselves or their spouse/partner:

Matthew J. Bassignani, MD (Test Author) is on the Advisory Board/Committee for Nuance and Fuji Medical Systems.
Vikram S. Dogra, MD (Consulting Editor) is the Editor of the Journal of Clinicl Imaging Science.
Andrej Lyshchik, MD, PhD is a consultant for Pfizer, Inc.
Dolores H. Pretorius, MD receives software support from GE Healthcare and Phillips Medical Systems.

Disclosure of Discussion of Non-FDA Approved Uses for Pharmaceutical Products and/or Medical Devices

The University of Virginia School of Medicine, as an ACCME provider, requires that all faculty presenters identify and disclose any off-label uses for pharmaceutical and medical device products. The University of Virginia School of Medicine recommends that each physician fully review all the available data on new products or procedures prior to clinical use.

TO ENROLL

To enroll in the Ultrasound Clinics Continuing Medical Education program, call customer service at 1-800-654-2452 or visit us online at www.theclinics.com/home/cme. The CME program is available to subscribers for an additional fee of $196.00.

Preface
Ultrasound in Obstetrics and Gynecology

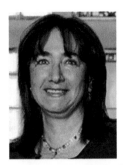

Phyllis Glanc, MD, FRCPC (C)
Guest Editor

This issue of *Ultrasound Clinics* on selected topics in Obstetrics and Gynecology has been a pleasure to edit. When one sits down to plan an *Ultrasound Clinics* on such a diverse topic, the challenge is to select the areas that will be of clinical relevance to the reader. We have been fortunate in having a diverse expert authorship including North America, Europe, and Israel. This diversity reflects some of the international differences in both the way we practice and the way we wish to practice in our field.

In the obstetrics section, we have looked at new and expanding views in fetal echocardiography as well as classic pitfalls that we may all experience in imaging of the second and third trimester. We have been fortunate to have our outstanding British colleagues contribute cutting edge sections on gestational trophoblastic disease and the role of ultrasound in the management of threatened miscarriage. The question of when to perform an anatomic fetal evaluation is explored in the article on early first-trimester anatomy. Although the debate may be ongoing, it has raised many interesting questions.

In the gynecology section, we have an excellent article on demystifying ovarian cysts in addition to a superb update on the use of color Doppler sonography in the pelvis. We are fortunate to have the authors of established guidelines on postmenopausal bleeding present a review of this topic for this issue. Pediatric gynecology, always a challenge for the adult imager, is presented in a concise fashion. The superb discussion of nongynecological causes of right lower quadrant pain, in particular that of bowel, has simplified what has traditionally been a challenging area for ultrasound imagers.

Hopefully after reading this issue of *Ultrasound Clinics*, the reader will have a perspective on some new and exciting directions in our field and solidify some practice models in their daily work. By extending our understanding and knowledge of ultrasound imaging, we can contribute to the campaigns of "Image Wisely and Gently," thus reducing radiation exposure where warranted.

Many thanks to the excellent work and support by the staff at Elsevier.

My sincere thanks and respect to the authors for their willingness to share their expertise in their respective fields.

Phyllis Glanc, MD, FRCPC (C)
Abdominal Imaging Division
Department of Medical Imaging
Department of Obstetrics & Gynecology
University of Toronto, 92 College Street
Toronto, ON M5G 1L4, Canada

Obstetrical Ultrasound Centre
Sunnybrook Health Science Centre
2075 Bayview Avenue
Toronto, ON M4N 3M5, Canada

E-mail address:
Phyllis.Glanc@sunnybrook.ca

Ultrasound Clin 7 (2012) xi
doi:10.1016/j.cult.2011.11.002
1556-858X/12/$ – see front matter

Fetal Echocardiography: The Four-Chamber View, the Outflow Tracts, and the Contribution of the Cardiac Arches

Alina Weissmann-Brenner, MD[a,b,*], Dolores H. Pretorius, MD[c], Reuven Achiron, MD[a,b], Liat Gindes, MD[a,b]

KEYWORDS

- Echocardiography • Cardiac arches • Outflow tracts
- Four-chamber view

The prenatal diagnosis of congenital heart disease (CHD) is of great consequence, due to its high incidence at birth of 4 to 8 per 1000 neonates, and elevated rates of neonatal mortality (20%–30%).[1,2] The prenatal diagnosis of CHD enables patients to be advised about the prognosis and the possible options of treatment. Karyotyping can be offered because of the strong association between cardiac defects and chromosomal abnormalities, including microdeletions.[3–5] Time and mode of delivery can be scheduled ahead, along with referral to tertiary centers for delivery. Patients can even choose to terminate the pregnancy when severe CHD is diagnosed at early stages. Furthermore, normal echocardiography may reassure high-risk patients (such as fetuses with increased nuchal translucency, family history of CHD, and pregestational diabetes).

Fetal cardiac examinations pose a challenge to sonographers, due to the complexity of the heart and the dependency on fetal position and maternal body characteristics. While many congenital heart lesions can be demonstrated prenatally, some anomalies are still difficult to diagnose in utero (ie, coarctation of aorta, atrial septal defect [ASD]).

Sonographic imaging of the fetal heart includes 2-dimensional (2D), 3-dimensional (3D), and 4-dimensional (4D) ultrasonography combined with application of color and pulsed Doppler. One advantage of 3D/4D ultrasonography is the ability to navigate the volume and to rotate it, thus demonstrating additional angles other than the original angle of acquisition; this postprocessing process can be performed at a different time and place and by different medical providers. The ability to diagnose cardiac malformations by 4D ultrasound volumes was

The authors have nothing to disclose.

[a] Department of Obstetrics and Gynecology, The Chaim Sheba Medical Center, Tel-Hashomer, Ramat Gan 52621, Israel

[b] Sackler Faculty of Medicine, Tel Aviv University, Ramat Aviv, PO Box 39040, Tel Aviv 69978, Israel

[c] UCSD Thornton Hospital, 9300 Campus Point Drive, 7756 La Jolla, CA 92037, USA

* Corresponding author. Department of Obstetrics and Gynecology, The Chaim Sheba Medical Center, Tel-Hashomer, Ramat Gan 52621, Israel.

E-mail address: alinabrenner@yahoo.com

Ultrasound Clin 7 (2012) 1–13

doi:10.1016/j.cult.2011.08.005

1556-858X/12/$ – see front matter © 2012 Elsevier Inc. All rights reserved

examined in a large collaborative study of leading centers from several countries. The sensitivity, specificity, positive and negative predictive values, and false-positive and false-negative rates for the identification of fetuses with CHD was 93%, 96%, 96%, 93%, 4.8%, and 6.8%, respectively.[6]

Cardiac examination of the 4-chamber view (4CV) enables detection of many major congenital heart abnormalities; however, it cannot identify all lesions. Several cardiac anomalies have a normal 4CV but an abnormal outflow tract or abnormal course, size, or spatial location of the great arteries (ie, transposition of the great arteries). Recognition of the ductus arteriosus, aortic arch, and superior vena cava (SVC) as well as the trachea in the views of the upper mediastinum is extremely helpful for complete cardiac assessment.[7,8]

The objective of this article is to assess the added value of the 3-vessel and trachea (3VT) view along with the cardiac arches in conjunction with the 4CV in fetal echocardiography.

CARDIAC EXAMINATION

Guidelines for the performance of fetal heart examinations have been published by the International Society of Ultrasound in Obstetrics and Gynecology,[9] and include 5 axial views: the situs, the 4CV, the left ventricle outflow tract, the right ventricle outflow tract, and the 3VT view (**Fig. 1**).

Situs and Axis

The fetal heart should be in the middle of the chest with the apex to the left, and the ventricular

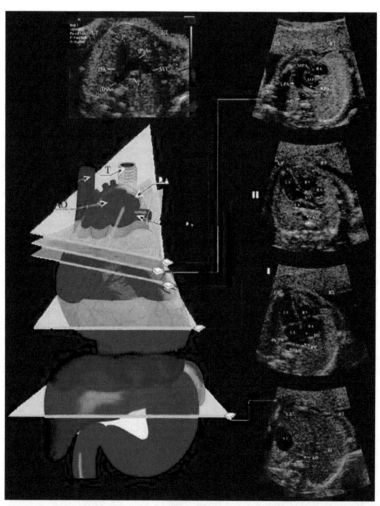

Fig. 1. The five axial views in the normal cardiac examination. In the lower image the situs is determined. The plane above is the 4-chamber view (4CV). More cephalic is the left and right outflow tract. The highest plane is the arches at the 3-vessel and trachea (3VT) view. (*From* Yagel S, Cohen SM, Achiron R. Examination of the fetal heart by five short-axis views: a proposed screening method for comprehensive cardiac evaluation. Ultrasound Obstet Gynecol 2001;368; with permission.)

septum should be at 45° from the midline; this is called levocardia. The presence of abnormal cardiac axis is associated with a substantial risk of congenital heart defects.[10,11] The term situs is used to define the position of asymmetric organs relative to the midline: lungs, liver, spleen, and stomach.[12] The position of the inferior vena cava (IVC) slightly anterior and to the right of the aorta can also be assessed for situs. The fetal heart should occupy one-third of thoracic area.[13]

Situs solitus is the normal arrangement of abdominal organs, with levocardia. The incidence of CHD is less than 1%. Situs inversus is a mirror-image location of the heart and abdominal viscera, and is almost always associated with dextrocardia. In this situation the incidence of CHD is 3% to 5%. Heterotaxy is a disorderly arrangement of organs and major blood vessels, in which the incidence of CHD is very high. An exception is isolated levocardia, in which the heart is in the normal levo position and the abdominal viscera are in dextroposition.[14]

The 4-Chamber View

Examination of the 4CV includes inspection of the atria, ventricles, interventricular septum, foramen ovale, interatrial septum, atrioventricular valves, and position of the descending aorta on the left. The two atria should be of equal size, with foramen ovale flap to the left, and at least 3 pulmonary veins should be seen entering the left atrium. In the normal heart, the atrial septum primum should be inspected and the two ventricles should be of equal size with normal cardiac walls, that is, without hypertrophy. The right ventricle includes the moderator band and the left ventricle forms the cardiac apex. The ventricular septum is intact.[13] Both atrioventricular valves open and move freely, the tricuspid valve positioned slightly closer to the apex than the mitral valve. The tricuspid valve has a septal leaflet whereas the mitral valve does not have a septal leaflet.

Anomalies that may be detected on the 4CV include muscle hypertrophy, abnormal chambers (hypoplastic heart, ventricular asymmetry, atrial asymmetry), abnormal valves (regurgitation or stenosis, Ebstein anomaly), and abnormal interventricular septum (ventricular septal defect [VSD], atrioventricular septal defect [AVSD]). Before making any diagnosis of an anomaly, one should be familiar with the artifacts. The explanation of cardiac artifacts is beyond the goals of this article; however, it is important to know that pseudo-VSD occurs when the ventricular septum is parallel to the ultrasound beam and pseudo-AVSD occurs when the septum is perpendicular to the ultrasound beam.

Left Ventricular Outflow Tract

The normal left ventricular outflow tract (LVOT) is composed of the aorta ascending from the left ventricle toward the right side, crossing the left main stem bronchus at the level of T5 thoracic vertebra, and descending left of the midline to the diaphragm. The normal branching pattern of the aortic arch includes the right innominate artery, which branches into the right common carotid and right subclavian arteries; the left common carotid artery; and the left subclavian artery. Anomalies of the outflow tracts and cardiac arches are discussed in the following sections.

Right Ventricular Outflow Tract

The normal right ventricular outflow tract (RVOT) is composed of the main pulmonary artery ascending from the right ventricle and branching to the right, and left pulmonary arteries and the ductus arteriosus. The ductus arteriosus connects the left pulmonary artery to the aorta distal to the left subclavian artery.

The Arches

An axial cephalic step from the 4CV reveals the 3VT view (**Fig. 2**). This view is a transverse one of the fetal upper mediastinum, demonstrating the oblique section of the main pulmonary artery and ductus arteriosus, cross section of the ascending aorta, and superior vena cava arranged in a straight line from the left anterior to the right posterior aspect of the mediastinum.[7] The main pulmonary artery is the largest of the 3 vessels, the ascending aorta is smaller by a factor of about 0.75, and the SVC the smallest (see the normograms in Ref.[15]). A V-shaped appearance of the great vessels is formed, with the left arm of the V representing the ductal arch and the right arm representing the aortic arch.[15,16] The blood vessels

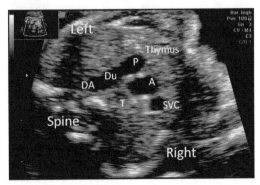

Fig. 2. Axial image of normal 3VT view. A, aortic arch; DA, descending aorta; Du, ductus arteriosus; P, pulmonary artery; SVC, superior vena cava; T, trachea.

demonstrate a linear growth during pregnancy.[17] The thymus can also be evaluated in the upper mediastinum axial plane, situated anteriorly in the midline.[18] Similarly, the innominate vein can be demonstrated passing anterior to the aorta horizontally. The cross section of the normal trachea reveals a hypoechoic round structure with echogenic borders located at the posterior part of the chest. The normal aortic arch is to the left of the trachea.[15] Demonstration of the location of the aortic arch in relation to the trachea is possible because the fetal airway is normally filled with fluid.[16]

Addition of Doppler to the 3VT view demonstrates that flow in the pulmonary artery and in the aorta is in the same direction, and the flow in the SVC is in the opposite direction (**Fig. 3**). Flow in the veins is at lower velocities than the arteries, therefore the pulse repetition frequency (PRF or scale velocity) should be reduced to demonstrate color in the SVC.

Embryologically, the aortic arches are a series of 6 paired embryologic vascular structures that give rise to the major arteries. The fourth left arch constitutes the arch of the aorta between the origin of the left carotid artery and the termination of the ductus arteriosus. The sixth left arch gives off the pulmonary arteries and forms the ductus arteriosus. According to a model described by Edwards[19] in 1948, two aortic arches connect the ascending and descending aorta, forming a complete vascular ring around the trachea and esophagus. Each aortic arch gives rise to a common carotid artery and a subclavian artery. Initially, right and left ducti arteriosi exist. Normally the left aortic arch and the left ductus persist, and regression of

the right arch occurs distal to the origin of the right subclavian artery and the right ductus arteriosus. The proximal part of the embryologic right aortic arch becomes the right innominate artery. Most aortic arch anomalies result from abnormal persistence of a part or parts that should have regressed, or abnormal regression of part or parts that should have persisted.[19,20]

The embryologic development of the venous system is more complex. It starts similarly with 3 pairs of symmetric bilateral vessels that completely or partially regress on one side. The cardinal veins become the vena cava and azygous veins, the vitaline veins develop into the portal system, and the umbilical veins connect the placental blood to the liver and heart of the fetus.[21–23]

In general, most of the arteries on the right side and most of the veins on the left side regress, whereas most arteries on the left side and most veins on the right side remain. Understanding the basic embryology as well as knowledge of the anatomy and the 3D multiplanar sections of the heart and great vessels are essential for the detection of malformations of the blood vessels.

4D VISUALIZATION OF THE OUTFLOW TRACTS AND ARCHES

The heart is a moving organ, therefore 3D analysis is insufficient. Two methods of 4D ultrasonography of the fetal heart are available: (1) real-time 4D and (2) spatiotemporal image correlation (STIC), in which multiple 3D volumes are acquired and the computer reorganizes them to a cine-loop of one cardiac cycle.[24–31] In the multiplanar display the screen is divided into 3 frames of 2D images or 2D clips that are perpendicular to each other; the axial, sagittal, and coronal planes of the organ may be demonstrated on the same screen. The cursor dot is located on the same location in all 3 planes, and can be moved. All the images can be rotated on 3 axes (X, Y, and Z) and also from front to back.

A good STIC acquisition allows the operator to scroll through the acquired volume from top to bottom along the original plane of acquisition and to obtain sequentially each of the 5 classic axial planes of fetal echocardiography, and any plane may be viewed at any time point throughout the reconstructed cardiac cycle loop. Visualization of the aortic and ductal arches as well as the venous return to the heart is best accomplished in volume data sets acquired using sagittal sweeps through the fetal chest.[24,27–29]

To obtain the sagittal aortic arch view from the gray-scale volume, the operator scrolls from the 4CV in a cephalad direction to the 3VT view and

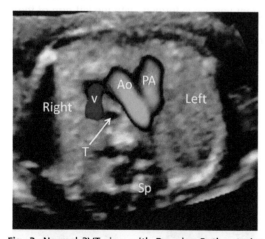

Fig. 3. Normal 3VT view with Doppler. Both arteries are in blue and the vein is in red. The right and left side of the fetus are annotated. Ao, aorta; PA, pulmonary artery; Sp, spine; T, trachea; V, superior vena cava.

puts the cursor dot on the aorta (the middle vessel in a normal heart). Working with sectional planes, the sagittal image of the aortic arch will be seen on the right image as a candy cane–shaped structure, giving rise to the head and neck vessels (**Fig. 4**A).

The ductal arch is demonstrated by moving the cursor dot of interest to the ductus arteriosus on the left image (A plane) (the vessel on the left in the normal heart) and straightening the vessel of interest along the vertical axis. The sagittal image of the ductal arch is on the right image (B plane) (see **Fig. 4**B).

Demonstration of the entrance of the veins to the right atrium on the sagittal plane can be achieved by moving the cursor dot of interest to the right atrium at the 4CV or to the SVC at the 3VT plane (the vessel on the right in the normal heart) (see **Fig. 4**C).

These views and manipulations can also be generated by acquiring volume data sets with color Doppler, power Doppler, or high-definition Doppler.

Using the B-flow technique in combination with 4D ultrasonography of the heart enables the examiner to demonstrate blood flow in the heart and the great vessels.[25] The combination of B-flow with STIC along with the creation of a rendered image allows for very sensitive demonstration of blood vessels and heart chambers (**Fig. 5**). Gindes and colleagues[30] demonstrated that inversion mode and B-flow were more informative than color Doppler imaging for detecting arch and systemic vein anomalies.

DIAGNOSTIC APPROACH TO ABNORMAL OUTFLOW TRACTS AND CARDIAC ARCHES

The prenatal diagnosis of cardiac outflow tracts and arch anomalies is challenging. Systematic evaluation of the normal and abnormal arches should include the following: number and size of vessels, their spatial arrangements, location of the vessels compared with the trachea, and the direction of blood flow through the vessels.

Abnormal Vessel Number

The first step in evaluation of the upper mediastinum vessels is to count the number of vessels in the 3VT view, and this should be done with gray-scale ultrasonography. In abnormal cases it is not always easy to diagnose the specific vessel, but counting the number narrows the differential diagnosis. The number of vessels can be normal, decreased, or increased.

Presence of Two Vessels

The presence of two vessels (one artery and one vein) in 3VT view is rare. The differential diagnosis of a single artery includes a true single artery (ie, truncus arteriosus), or two arteries with demonstration of only one of them. *Truncus arteriosus is*

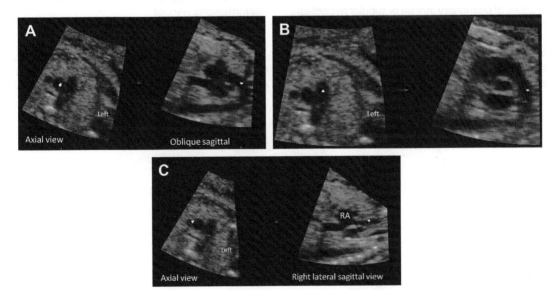

Fig. 4. Ultrasound volume presented as 2-dimensional images that are perpendicular to each other. The white dot is in the same places in the image pairs. (*A*) The white dot is on the aortic arch. (*B*) Moving the dot to the left vessel and straightening the vessel along the vertical line will demonstrate the ductal arch. (*C*) Moving the dot to the right on the axial plane will change the sagittal plane so the superior (*white dot location*) and inferior vena cava are seen entering the right atrium. RA, right atrium.

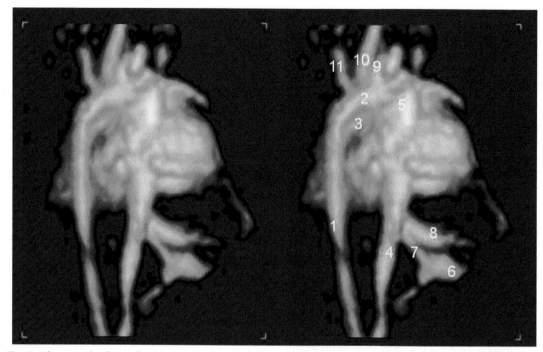

Fig. 5. Ultrasound volume that was acquired with B-flow and spatiotemporal image correlation (STIC) technologies of normal fetus at 23 gestational weeks. Same image, with the image on the right labeled. 1, aorta; 2, aortic arch; 3, ductal arch; 4, inferior vena cava; 5, superior vena cava; 6, umbilical vein; 7, ductus venosus; 8, hepatic vein; 9, right brachiocephalic artery; 10, left common carotid artery; 11, left subclavian artery.

a rare cardiac anomaly (5–15:100,000 live births) in which only one artery exits the heart. It is usually associated with valve anomalies.

A stenotic artery may not be seen, for example in cases of pulmonary atresia or tubular hypoplasia of aorta, or in cases of severe tetralogy of Fallot (TOF) with a small pulmonary artery. Another situation in which one of the vessels is not demonstrated in the 3VT view is when the spatial arrangement of the vessels is parallel and one of the arteries lies on top of the other. In this case the axial plane fails to demonstrate both arteries and only the sagittal view will demonstrate the abnormal anatomy, that is, in TOF and conotruncal malformations (**Fig. 6**).

Conotruncal Malformations

Conotruncal malformations include truncus arteriosus, TOF, pulmonary atresia with ventricular

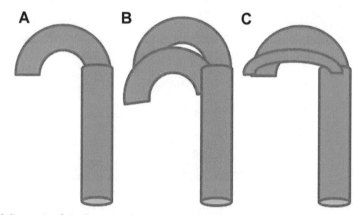

Fig. 6. Differential diagnosis of single artery demonstrated by ultrasound. (*A*) Only one vessel is seen (as in truncal anomaly). (*B*) Both vessels exist but their special place is one above the other, so in the axial plane only one vessel is demonstrated. (*C*) One of the vessels is very narrow and is not demonstrated easily.

septal defect, interrupted aortic arch, and transposition of the great arteries (TGA) and right aortic arch (RAA). Patients with these cardiac defects are frequently found to have a common microdeletion on chromosome 22, the so-called monosomy 22q11.2.[32]

Demonstration of 4 Vessels

Demonstration of 4 vessels in the 3VT view is usually caused by an extra vein but may also be related to an additional artery. Two veins may be seen in cases of bilateral SVC or persistent left SVC (PLSVC), in aberrant right subclavian artery (ARSA), and in partial anomalous pulmonary venous connection. If the extra vessel is an artery then double aortic arch is suspected. When 4 vessels are demonstrated in the 3VT view, the nature of all vessels needs verification. The examiner needs to try to identify the aorta, the pulmonary artery, and the SVC, their spatial arrangement, and the difference from the normal arrangement, and must try to trace the additional vessel to its source and to its destination. In general, any vessel crossing behind the trachea should be considered as an abnormal aberrant vessel.

Persistent left superior vena cava

The presence of a PLSVC can be attributed to the persistence of the proximal part of the left anterior cardinal vein. The PLSVC runs between the left atrial appendage and the left pulmonary veins, and almost always runs behind the left atrium and enters the right atrium through the orifice of an enlarged coronary sinus. In 65% of cases the innominate vein is absent or small. In approximately 8% of patients the PLSVC drains directly into the left atrium. Its prevalence is 0.2% of the general population, and occurs in 9% of patients with CHD.[33] PLSVC as an isolated finding has no clinical impact because the systemic venous blood continues to return to the right atrium via the coronary sinus, and usually there is a normal right SVC. However, it may be associated with CHD, specifically heterotaxy syndromes.[33] The 3VT view demonstrates a fourth vessel to the left of the pulmonary trunk and arterial duct. In the 4CV an enlarged coronary sinus is seen (**Figs. 7 and 8**).

Aberrant right subclavian artery

ARSA arises from the normal left-sided aortic arch and crosses the mediastinum from left to right, behind the esophagus and trachea. It is caused by interruption of the dorsal segment of the right arch between the right carotid artery and right subclavian artery with regression of the right ductus arteriosus. Rarely, the right ductus may persist between the ARSA and the right pulmonary artery,

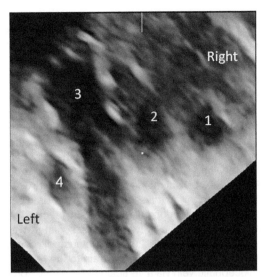

Fig. 7. Abnormal 3VT view. Four vessels are present instead of 3. 1, superior vena cava (*right*); 2, aorta; 3, pulmonary artery; 4, left persistent superior vena cava.

forming a complete vascular ring. In this situation, the proximal part of the aberrant artery is a wide channel carrying the blood from the ductus into the descending aorta. After birth, with closure of the ductus, the dilated proximal part persists as the aortic diverticulum of Kommerell.[13,34] ARSA is the most common aortic arch anomaly, with an incidence of 0.5% to 2%.[28] In general it is isolated, but may be associated with other cardiovascular anomalies, such as coarctation of the aorta, patent ductus arteriosus, intracardiac defects, anomalous pulmonary artery circulation, and carotid or vertebral artery anomalies. ARSA may be

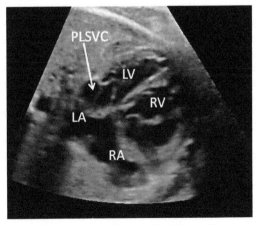

Fig. 8. Four-chamber view of the heart. The arrow points to a circle representing the entrance of the persistent left superior vena cava (PLSVC) to the coronary sinus. LA, left atrium; LV, left ventricle; RA, right atrium; RV, right ventricle.

associated with trisomy 21 and microdeletion 22q11 chromosome (up to 37% of cases in the studies of Zalel and colleagues and Chaoui and colleagues[35–37]).

Partial anomalous pulmonary venous connection

Partial anomalous pulmonary venous connection (PAPVR) has a prevalence of 0.4% to 0.7%. At least one pulmonary vein drains to a location other than the left atrium, usually affecting the right lung and resulting in a left to right shunt, similar to an ASD, VSD, or patent ductus arteriosus. PAPVR most commonly involves the anomalous drainage of the right superior pulmonary vein to the right atrium or SVC, and is frequently associated with a sinus venosus ASD. Left anomalous pulmonary venous structures commonly drain to the left brachiocephalic vein via a vertical vein or to the coronary sinus. In this condition the 4CV shows the right lower pulmonary vein connecting to the left atrium. Left pulmonary veins cannot be traced back to the left atrium. The 3VT view may show an additional vessel (vertical vein) on the left side of the main pulmonary artery. The vertical vein collects the left pulmonary veins and connects them to the innominate vein.[38]

Double aortic arch

Double aortic arch represents a persistence of both right and left fourth aortic arches that form a complete vascular ring around the trachea and esophagus. The left arch is anterior while the posterior right arch courses to the left behind the esophagus, where it joins the left arch. The descending aorta is usually on the left side. The common carotid and subclavian arteries arise separately from each arch and are usually symmetrically arranged. The right arch is larger in approximately 75% of cases. The left ductus is patent in the majority of cases. The 3VT view shows that the left and right aortic arches form a complete circle around the trachea. This anomaly is the most common cause of a complete vascular ring. Associated congenital heart anomalies are found in approximately 20% of cases (Fig. 9).[7,39,40]

The presence of 3 vessels in the 3VT view rules out the previously mentioned anomalies, yet the examiner needs to verify the exact arrangement and alignment of the vessels. Once again, each vessel needs to be traced to its origin and to its destination in order to establish which vessel it is.

Abnormal Vessel Arrangement

Abnormal vessel arrangement refers to a change in the left to right organization of the 3 vessels.

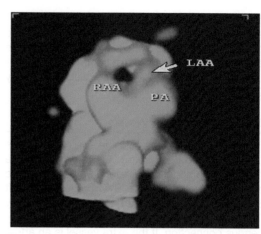

Fig. 9. Double aortic arch demonstrated from a volume, acquired using STIC with gray-scale imaging and postprocessing with inversion mode. Both arches create a ring around the trachea. PA, pulmonary artery; LAA, left aortic arch; RAA, right aortic arch.

The normal aortic arch is on the left of the trachea, with the descending aorta being on the left anterior aspect of the vertebral body. The left- or right-sidedness of the aortic arch refers to the position of the aortic arch relative to the trachea.

Right aortic arch

The RAA is a relatively common anomaly, with a prevalence of approximately 0.05%. It is formed with regression of the left aortic arch distal to the origin of the left subclavian artery. RAA gives rise to the left innominate, right carotid, and right subclavian arteries in sequence, which is a mirror image of a normal left aortic arch. Usually a left ductus is patent. This variant does not form a vascular ring or sling. It is almost always associated with CHD, most commonly cyanotic CHD, especially TOF with or without pulmonary atresia and truncus arteriosus. In the 3VT view a U-shaped configuration is seen, with the trachea located between the arms of the U (Figs. 10 and 11).[13,34,39,40] When the RAA is associated with TOF the patent ductus tends to be small, and the blood flow through it can be reversed or bidirectional.

Abnormal Size of Vessels

Small ascending aorta and large main pulmonary artery

The size of the vessels reflects the amount of blood passing through them. A small ascending aorta and large main pulmonary artery reflect diversion of blood flow from the left side to the right side, and may be attributed to anomalies in the left ventricle or the aorta, such as hypoplastic left heart, critical aortic stenosis, coarctation of aorta, and interruption of the aortic arch (Fig. 12).

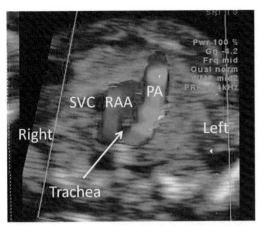

Fig. 10. Two-dimensional imaging on axial plane of right aortic arch (RAA). The RAA and the pulmonary artery (PA) create a U-shape around the trachea. SVC, superior vena cava.

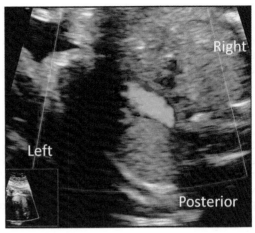

Fig. 12. A small ascending aorta and large main pulmonary artery in a 26-week fetus. This patient also has large outlet ventricular septal defect, and postnatal diagnosis was interruption of aortic arch type B.

Hypoplasia of left heart The birth incidence of hypoplasia of left heart (HLH) is 0.1 to 0.25 per 1000 live births, and comprises 7% of all CHD.[34] The 4CV plane reveals a small, thick-walled hyperechoic left ventricle with or secondary to mitral atresia or hypoplasia. The outflow of the left

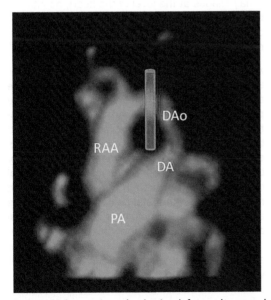

Fig. 11. Right aortic arch obtained from ultrasound volume acquired by B-flow and STIC. The trachea was drawn (brown vertical cylinder) as an overlay on the image. It cannot be demonstrated with the B-flow technique. RAA, right aortic arch; DAo, descending aorta; DA, ductus arteriosus; PA, pulmonary artery.

ventricle is scarcely demonstrated. In the 3VT view the aorta is small or not visible.

Critical aortic stenosis The birth incidence of critical aortic stenosis is 6 in 1000 live births, and it comprises 3% to 5% of all CHD. In the 4CV the left ventricle may appear echogenic and poorly contracting, the mitral valve is patent, and the aortic valve stenotic.[41] In some cases the left ventricle may appear normal or dilated and eventually may progress to HLH.[42] In the 3VT view the aorta is small. In severe cases, as a result of the high pressure in the left ventricle, the mitral valve is damaged and mitral regurgitation may occur. The direction of flow through the foramen ovale is toward the right ventricle. Inverted flow in the aortic arch indicates a poor prognosis.

Coarctation of aorta This anomaly accounts for approximately 7% of all live births with CHD. It is usually associated with other cardiac lesions including VSD, patent ductus arteriosus, and bicuspid aortic valve.[43] The 4CV shows right-sided dominance in chamber size. The flap valve of the fossa ovalis bulges toward the right atrium. The aortic-arch view often shows a small aortic arch and isthmus and an abnormal flow pattern on color Doppler imaging. This lesion may be extremely subtle on fetal imaging and will not be identified in many cases.

Interruption of aortic arch
This rare congenital anomaly (2:100,000 live births) associated in 50% of cases with deletion in chromosome 22 and DiGeorge syndrome, and

characterized by the separation between the ascending and descending aorta. Additional cardiovascular anatomic defects are found in up to 98% of cases, especially patent ductus arteriosus. Sonographic findings include enlarged pulmonary artery, VSD, and hypoplastic aortic arch.[44]

Small main pulmonary artery and large ascending aorta

Small main pulmonary artery and large ascending aorta reflects diversion of blood from the right side to the left as a result of anomalies in the right ventricle and pulmonary artery, such as TOF, pulmonary stenosis, Ebstein malformation, and congenital diaphragmatic hernia.

Tetralogy of Fallot TOF occurs in 1 of 3600 live births and comprises 3.5% of all liveborns with CHD. The 4CV reveals a large VSD. The views of the outflow tracts are crucial for the diagnosis of TOF. Leftward, anterior, and superior deviation of the outlet septum causes subpulmonary outflow tract narrowing and an outlet type of VSD, and subpulmonary and pulmonary stenosis. In the 3VT view the main pulmonary artery is small and may be difficult to identify, and the ascending aorta dilated.[32]

Pulmonary atresia or critical stenosis with or without VSD Pulmonary stenosis comprises 10% of CHD, and is often seen with other cardiac anomalies. The ascending aorta is more anteriorly located in relation to the main pulmonary artery. The pulmonary artery is slightly smaller than the ascending aorta. The ductal arch view with color Doppler may show a left to right shunt across the ductus. In cases with intact ventricular septum, the 4CV shows severe hypoplasia of the right ventricular cavity and thickened right ventricular free wall.

Ebstein malformation In this rare cardiac anomaly (1:20,000 live births, comprising 1% of all CHD), the leaves of the tricuspid valves are displaced and stiff. The 4CV demonstrates enlarged right atrium with the tricuspid valve closer to the apex, with tricuspid insufficiency, and in severe cases pulmonary stenosis. Additional cardiac anomalies include VSD, ASD, TOF, TGA, and coarctation of aorta. In the 3VT view the aorta is larger than the pulmonary artery.

In cases of congenital diaphragmatic hernia (1:2500 live births) the diameter of the main pulmonary artery may be smaller than in normal fetuses, because of a decrease in blood flow in the branches of the pulmonary artery due to pressure from the herniated viscera. Indeed, measurements of the pulmonary artery are used to predict pulmonary hypoplasia and outcome in these cases.[31,45,46]

Dilated main pulmonary artery and dilated ascending aorta

Dilated main pulmonary artery may be caused by both pulmonary valve stenosis and regurgitation. Dilated ascending aorta may be caused by aortic valve stenosis due to poststenotic dilatation, in aortic regurgitation, or rarely in cases with Marfan syndrome. Achiron and colleagues[16] described normograms for fetal aorta and pulmonary artery, and Schneider and colleagues[45] developed Z-scores for the aorta and pulmonary artery.

Dilated superior vena cava

Dilated SVC may be caused by interruption of the IVC with azygos continuation, anomalous pulmonary venous connection, right-sided heart failure, and vein of Galen aneurysm. In any case of dilated SVC, the sonographer should try to demonstrate the drainage of all 4 pulmonary veins.

Interruption of the IVC with azygos continuation This anomaly may be isolated, though frequently it is associated with cardiac anomalies or situs anomalies, most frequently polysplenia syndrome (85%). The azygos vein is situated posterior to the aorta. The sonographic signs include a vessel parallel to the aorta (slightly smaller in caliber) on sagittal views, double vessel sign on transverse (axial) images at the level of the heart, no intrahepatic portion of the IVC, normal hepatic veins and ductus venosus, and, in cardiosplenic syndromes, cardiac and intra-abdominal abnormalities.[12,47,48]

Anomalous pulmonary venous connection Anomalous pulmonary venous connection is a rare anomaly (7:1,000,000 live births) in which the pulmonary veins are drained to the right side of the heart while the left atrium receives oxygenated blood through the foramen ovale and ASD.[32] It is essential to make this diagnosis prenatally because of its lethal consequences. The abnormal drainage could be through a vertical vein, which may be found in the fetal chest or abdomen. This anomaly can be complete or partial. Additional anomalies are ASD and heterotaxy syndrome. Sonographic findings include enlargement of right atrium and right ventricle, ASD, and improper venous drainage to the heart.

Abnormal Vessel Alignment

Abnormal vessel alignment refers to the 3 vessels not arranged in a straight line, yet their left to right order is preserved. The most common abnormal alignment is caused by anterior displacement of ascending aorta with small main pulmonary artery.

This may be seen in TOF, and in double-outlet right ventricle with subpulmonary stenosis.

In TOF the ascending aorta is dilated and displaced anteriorly and to the right, whereas the main pulmonary artery is smaller and displaced posteriorly.

Double-outlet right ventricle with subpulmonary stenosis is a rare cardiac anomaly (3:100,000 live births), with 3 variants: right aorta parallel to the pulmonary artery, right aorta displaced anterior to the pulmonary artery, and anterior left aorta. VSD is present in the 4CV.

Posterior displacement of small ascending aorta is seen in severe cases of obstruction of the left side of the heart, such as hypoplastic left heart syndrome and interruption of the aortic arch.

Side-by-side relationship with small ascending aorta is seen in double-outlet right ventricle with subaortic stenosis, and complete transposition with subaortic stenosis.

Side-by-side relationship with the same arterial size is seen in double-outlet right ventricle and in TGA.

Transposition of the great arteries

The incidence of TGA is 1 in 2000 live births, and it comprises 5% of CHD.[32,37] There are two variants:

1. *D-transposition/complete TGA*. Aorta arises from the right ventricle and pulmonary artery from the left ventricle. Two separated blood flows are created.
2. *L-transposition/corrected TGA*. A rare type in which the right atrium is connected to the left ventricle from which the pulmonary artery derives, and the left atrium connects to the right ventricle from which the aorta derives. In this type there is a connection between the pulmonary and the systemic circulation.

Sonographic findings include parallel position of the aorta and the pulmonary artery. The aorta derives from the right ventricle and is anterior to the pulmonary artery that derives from the left ventricle. Associated anomalies are VSD, ASD, pulmonary stenosis, and arrhythmias. Most cases of complete TGA have the aorta right anterior to the pulmonary artery, whereas most cases with corrected TGA have the aorta left anterior to the pulmonary artery. VSD is found in 40% of complete TGA and in 60% to 70% of corrected TGA.

SUMMARY

The systematic sonographic evaluation of the fetal heart with emphasis on the outflow tract and arches demands understanding of the embryologic models and the possible pitfalls causing the different anomalies. The authors believe that the 3VT and sagittal aortic arch views are necessary to complete a fetal cardiac assessment. Abnormal number, arrangement, size, and alignment are indicators of anomalies. Abnormal position of the descending aorta, absence of the normal V-shaped confluence of the ductal and aortic arches, a gap between the ascending aorta and main pulmonary artery in the 3VT view, and an abnormal vessel behind the trachea with or without a U-shaped vascular loop or ring around the trachea are all clues aiding in the differential diagnosis of cardiac anomalies.

Careful sonographic cardiac evaluation may improve prenatal diagnosis of CHD, making early postnatal management optimal.

REFERENCES

1. Hoffman JI, Kaplan S. The incidence of congenital heart disease. J Am Coll Cardiol 2002;39:1890–900.
2. Hoffman JI. Incidence of congenital heart disease: I. Postnatal incidence. Pediatr Cardiol 1995;16:103–13.
3. McAuliffe FM, Trines J, Nield LE, et al. Early fetal echocardiography—a reliable prenatal diagnosis tool. Am J Obstet Gynecol 2005;193:1253–9.
4. Weiner Z, Lorber A, Shalev E. Diagnosis of congenital cardiac defects between 11 and 14 weeks' gestation in high risk population. J Ultrasound Med 2002;21:23–9.
5. Weiner Z, Weizman B, Beloosesky R, et al. Fetal cardiac scanning performed immediately following an abnormal nuchal translucency examination. Prenat Diagn 2008;28:934–8.
6. Espinoza J, Lee W, Comstock C, et al. Collaborative study on 4-dimensional echocardiography for the diagnosis of fetal heart defects: the COFEHD study. J Ultrasound Med 2010;29(11):1573–80.
7. Yoo SJ, Lee YH, Kim SH. Three vessel view of the fetal upper mediastinum: an easy means of detecting abnormalities of the ventricular outflow tracts and great arteries during obstetric screening. Ultrasound Obstet Gynecol 1997;9:173–82.
8. Yagel S, Arbel R, Anteby EY, et al. The three vessels and trachea view (3VT) in fetal cardiac scanning. Ultrasound Obstet Gynecol 2002;20:340–5.
9. International Society of Ultrasound in Obstetrics & Gynecology. Cardiac screening examination of the fetus: guidelines for performing the 'basic' and 'extended basic' cardiac scan. Ultrasound Obstet Gynecol 2006;27(1):107–13.
10. Shipp TD, Bromley B, Hornberger LK, et al. Levorotation of the fetal cardiac axis: a clue for the presence of congenital heart disease. Obstet Gynecol 1995;85(1):97–102.
11. Sinkovskaya E, Horton S, Berkley EM, et al. Defining the fetal cardiac axis between 11 + 0 and 14 + 6

weeks of gestation: experience with 100 consecutive pregnancies. Ultrasound Obstet Gynecol 2010; 36(6):676–81.

12. Winer-Muram HT, Tonkin IL. The spectrum of heterotaxic syndromes. Radiol Clin North Am 1989;27(6): 1147–70.

13. Lee W, Allan L, Carvalho JS, et al, ISUOG Fetal Echocardiography Task Force. ISUOG consensus statement: what constitutes a fetal echocardiogram? Ultrasound Obstet Gynecol 2008;32(2):239–42.

14. Gindes L, Hegesh J, Barkai G, et al. Isolated levocardia: Prenatal diagnosis, clinical significance and literature review. J Ultrasound Med 2007;26(3):361–5.

15. Zalel Y, Wiener Y, Gamzu R, et al. The three-vessel and tracheal view of the fetal heart: an in utero sonographic evaluation. Prenat Diagn 2004;24(3):174–8.

16. Achiron R, Rotstein Z, Heggesh J, et al. Anomalies of the fetal aortic arch: a novel sonographic approach to in utero diagnosis. Ultrasound Obstet Gynecol 2002;20:553–7.

17. Achiron R, Golan-Porat N, Gabbay U, et al. In utero ultrasonographic measurements of fetal aortic and pulmonary artery diameters during the first half of gestation. Ultrasound Obstet Gynecol 1998;11(3): 180–4.

18. Zalel Y, Gamzu R, Mashiach S, et al. The development of the fetal thymus: an in utero sonographic evaluation. Prenat Diagn 2002;22(2):114–7.

19. Edwards JE. Anomalies of the derivatives of the aortic arch system. Med Clin North Am 1948;32:925–48.

20. Edwards JE. Vascular rings and slings. In: Moller JH, Neal WE, Norwalk CT, editors. Fetal, neonatal and infant cardiac disease. Norwalk (CT): Appleton&Lange; 1990. p. 745–54.

21. Fasouliotis SJ, Achiron R, Kivilevitch Z, et al. The human fetal venous system: normal embryologic, anatomic, and physiologic characteristics and developmental abnormalities. J Ultrasound Med 2002;21(10):1145–58.

22. Cherian SB, Ramesh BR, Madhyastha S. Persistent left superior vena cava. Clin Anat 2006;19:561–5.

23. Peltier J, Destrieux C, Desme J, et al. The persistent left superior vena cava: anatomical study, pathogenesis and clinical considerations. Surg Radiol Anat 2006;28:206–10.

24. Sklansky M, Miller D, Devore G, et al. Prenatal screening for congenital heart disease using real-time three-dimensional echocardiography and a novel 'sweep volume' acquisition technique. Ultrasound Obstet Gynecol 2005;25(5):435–43.

25. Yagel S, Cohen SM, Shapiro I, et al. 3D and 4D ultrasound in fetal cardiac scanning: a new look at the fetal heart. Ultrasound Obstet Gynecol 2007;29:81–95.

26. Sklansky MS, Nelson TR, Strachan M, et al. Real-time three dimensional fetal echocardiography: initial feasibility study. J Ultrasound Med 1999;18: 745–52.

27. Yagel S, Benachi A, Bonnet D, et al. Rendering in fetal cardiac scanning: the intracardiac septa and the coronal atrioventricular valve planes. Ultrasound Obstet Gynecol 2006;28:266–74.

28. DeVore GR, Polanco B, Sklansky MS, et al. The 'spin' technique: a new method for examination of the fetal outflow tracts using three-dimensional ultrasound. Ultrasound Obstet Gynecol 2004;24(1):72–82.

29. DeVore GR, Falkensammer P, Sklansky MS, et al. Spatio-temporal image correlation (STIC): new technology for evaluation of the fetal heart. Ultrasound Obstet Gynecol 2003;22(4):380–7.

30. Gindes L, Hegesh J, Weisz B, et al. Three and four dimensional ultrasound: a novel method for evaluating fetal cardiac anomalies. Prenat Diagn 2009; 29(7):645–53.

31. Nelson TR, Pretorius DH, Sklansky M, et al. Three-dimensional echocardiographic evaluation of fetal heart anatomy and function: acquisition, analysis and display. J Ultrasound Med 1996;15:1–9.

32. Yoo SJ, Jaeggi EJ. Ultrasound evaluation of the fetal heart. In: Callen PW, editor. Ultrasonography in obstetrics and gynecology. 5th edition. Philadelphia (PA): Elsevier; 2008. p. 511–67.

33. Galindo A, Gutherrez-Larraya F, Escribano D, et al. Clinical significance of left superior vena cava diagnosed in fetal life. Ultrasound Obstet Gynecol 2007; 30:151–61.

34. Turkvatan A, Buyukbayraktar FG, Olcer T, et al. Congenital anomalies of the aortic arch: evaluation with the use of multidetector computed tomography. Korean J Radiol 2009;10(2):176–84, 34.

35. Zalel Y, Achiron R, Yagel S, et al. Fetal aberrant right subclavian artery in normal and down syndrome fetuses. Ultrasound Obstet Gynecol 2008;31:25–9, 35.

36. Chaoui R, Heling KS, Sarioglu N, et al. Aberrant right subclavian artery as a new cardiac sign in second and third trimester fetuses with down syndrome. Am J Obstet Gynecol 2005;192:257–63.

37. Dillman JR, Yarram SG, Hernandez RJ. Imaging of pulmonary venous developmental anomalies. AJR Am J Roentgenol 2009;192:1272–85.

38. Yoo SJ, Bradely T, Jaeggi E. Aortic arch anomalies. In: Yagel S, Silverman NH, Gembruch U, editors. Fetal cardiology. 2nd edition. New York: Informa Healthcare; 2009. p. 329–42.

39. Simpson JM. Hypoplastic left heart. Ultrasound Obstet Gynecol 2000;15:271–8.

40. Mäkikallio K, McElhinney DB, Levine JC, et al. Fetal aortic valve stenosis and the evolution of hypoplastic left heart syndrome: patient selection for fetal intervention. Circulation 2006;113:1401–5.

41. Rosenthal E. Coarctation of the aorta from fetus to adult: curable condition or lifelong disease process? Heart 2005;91:1495–502.

42. Sokol J, Bohn D, Lacro RV, et al. Fetal pulmonary artery diameters and their association with lung

hypoplasia and postnatal outcome in congenital diaphragmatic hernia. Am J Obstet Gynecol 2002; 186(5):1085–90.

43. Rollins RC, Acherman RJ, Castillo WJ, et al. Aorta larger than pulmonary artery in the fetal 3-vessel view. Obstet Gynecol Surv 2009;64(6):372–4.

44. Dillman JR, Yarram SG, D'Amico AR, et al. Interrupted aortic arch: spectrum of MRI findings. AJR Am J Roentgenol 2008;190(6):1467–74.

45. Schneider C, McCrindle BW, Carvalho JS, et al. Development of Z-scores for fetal cardiac dimensions from echocardiography. Ultrasound Obstet Gynecol 2005;26:599–605.

46. Geley TE, Unsinn KM, Auckenthaler TM, et al. Azygos continuation of the inferior vena cava: sonographic demonstration of the renal artery ventral to the azygos vein as a clue to diagnosis. AJR Am J Roentgenol 1999;172:1659–62.

47. Sheley RC, Nyberg DA, Kapur R. Azygous continuation of the interrupted inferior vena cava: a clue to prenatal diagnosis of the cardiosplenic syndromes. J Ultrasound Med 1995;14: 381–7.

48. Skinner J, Hornung T, Rumball E. Transposition of the great arteries: from fetus to adult. Heart 2008; 94(9):1227–35.

Mistakes to Avoid in the Second and Third Trimesters: Fetal Measurements and Anatomy

Mary C. Frates, MD

KEYWORDS

- Fetal • Survey • Measurement • Anatomy

Obstetric ultrasonography is nearly universally used to evaluate the fetus for proper growth and to search for congenital anomalies. The American College of Radiology/American College of Obstetricians and Gynecologists/American Institute of Ultrasound in Medicine guidelines for the performance of obstetric sonography[1] outline the images that should be obtained in the second and third trimester, and many textbooks provide detailed instructions on how to obtain such images. However, the practice of obstetric sonography is full of challenges, and each patient and fetus is different from the prior. This article attempts to define and explain some common pitfalls that can occur when measuring the fetus and performing the fetal survey.

MEASUREMENTS

Accurate measurements of the fetus in the second and third trimesters are critical for the confirmation of a healthy ongoing pregnancy. Appropriate fetal growth is extremely reassuring for the physician and patient, whereas inappropriate growth indicates the need for additional evaluation, monitoring, and possible early intervention (delivery). For each fetal measurement, rules have been established to help ensure uniformity. Fetal size

and weight can be estimated using published tables of head, abdomen, and femur measurements or by using a variety of computer programs. For the fetal weight estimate to be as accurate as possible, the measurements used should be obtained using a standard technique. Many sources are available to the imager to learn proper measurement techniques.[2] It is critically important for the sonographer/sonologist to be thoroughly familiar with the standard techniques (know the rules), but it is just as important for the imager to follow the rules. This section discusses common mistakes that can occur while measuring the fetus.

For measurement of the biparietal diameter (BPD), calipers are placed on the skull rather than the skin surfaces and are placed on the leading edge of both near and far skull surfaces. The fetal head measurement must be obtained in a true axial plane. An off-axis plane causes the BPD to be over-measured or undermeasured. An off-axis or tilted image can be recognized when the midline falx is off center or when the paired thalami are not clearly visualized or are not located in the center of the fetal head. If the occipitofrontal diameter (OFD) is under-measured, a brachycephalic head is seen that is overly rounded. If the OFD is overmeasured, a dolichocephalic or flattened head shape is created. Common errors include not using the leading

The author has nothing to disclose.
Department of Radiology, Harvard Medical School, Brigham and Women's Hospital, 75 Francis Street, Boston, MA 02115, USA
E-mail address: mfrates@partners.org

Ultrasound Clin 7 (2012) 15–31
doi:10.1016/j.cult.2011.08.004
1556-858X/12/$ – see front matter © 2012 Elsevier Inc. All rights reserved.

edge of both the near and far skull as the caliper placement site as well as including the posterior fossa on the OFD image (**Fig. 1**).

The abdominal diameter measurement can also be challenging, particularly because the size of the fetus increases toward the end of pregnancy. Calipers must be placed at the skin surface where the skin meets amniotic fluid. This interface can be particularly difficult to identify in cases of overlapping fetal parts, placenta, or low levels of amniotic fluid or oligohydramnios or in patients with a large body habitus. One clue to assist in identifying the skin surface is to note the amount of echogenic subcutaneous fat in the fetus in a region where a good interface is present. The same amount of fat should be present around the entire abdomen, giving some hint as to the approximate location of the remaining skin surfaces. Another common mistake is to mark a rib as the skin surface. The skin is typically several millimeters away from the echogenic rib in the third trimester. The abdominal diameter should be measured on a true axial image, with the stomach and intrahepatic umbilical

vein both present on the image. As a general rule, fetal kidneys and lung bases do not appear on a true axial abdominal image. The perpendicular measurements of the abdominal wall should be within 10 mm of each other; this helps ensure a more accurate rounded shape of the abdomen rather than oval. If the imager uses too much pressure on the maternal abdominal wall, the amniotic fluid surrounding the fetus will be displaced to the sides and the fetal abdomen can be compressed into an oval shape. The solution in this situation is to reduce the transducer pressure and allow fluid to surround the fetal abdomen. In general, abdominal measurements should not be obtained when the fetus is prone. The fetal spine obscures the distal skin edge as well as the internal landmarks of the abdomen. In this situation, the solution is to image the fetus from one side or the other of the maternal abdomen or to roll the patient to image the fetus from the side (**Fig. 2**). When struggling, remember that a round shape is best and, even without all landmarks, is likely to be more accurate than an oblique image.

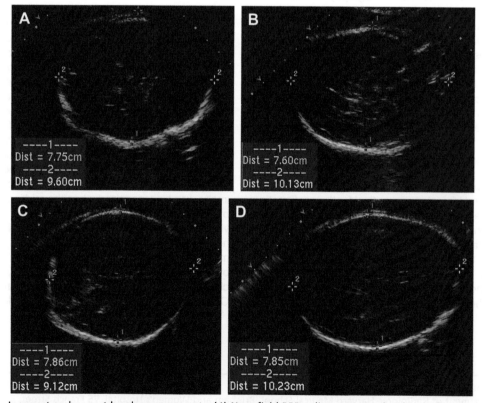

Fig. 1. Incorrect and correct head measurements. (*A*) Near-field BPD calipers are on the skin surface, instead of the leading edge of the skull. The posterior fossa is included on the image. (*B*) BPD calipers are correctly placed, but orbits are included on the image. (*C*) The posterior fossa is included on the image, and the head shape is too round. (*D*) Correct imaging plane and caliper placement. (© M.C. Frates. All Rights Reserved.)

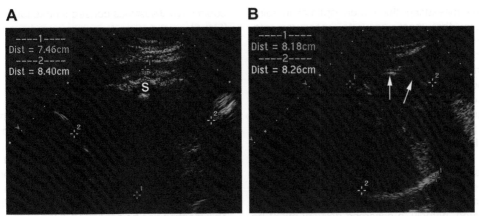

Fig. 2. Correct and incorrect abdominal diameter measurements. (*A*) Incorrect measurement. Fetus is prone, and shadowing spine (S) obscures the anterior abdominal wall skin surface and intra-abdominal anatomy. The lateral skin surfaces are obscured by fetal parts. The measurements are 10 mm apart. (*B*) Correct measurement technique. Same fetus, with mother rolled onto her side. Fetal skin surfaces and landmarks are now visible, and measurements are within 1 mm of each other. Note echogenic rib (*arrows*) deep to echogenic subcutaneous fat. (© M.C. Frates. All Rights Reserved.)

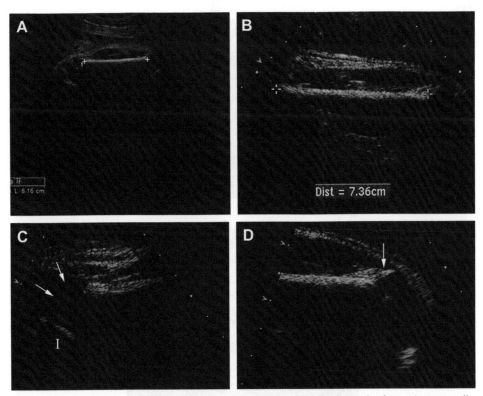

Fig. 3. Correct and incorrect femur measurements. (*A*) Depth is set too high, so the femur is too small, and the landmarks of the femur cannot be clearly identified. (*B*) Correct measurement. Femur is horizontal to the sound wave and fills the screen. (*C*) The proximal femur, with hypoechoic femoral head (*arrows*) (I, ilium). (*D*) The distal femoral point (*arrow*), an echogenic structure with no anatomic correlate that should not be included when measuring the femur. (© M.C. Frates. All Rights Reserved.)

When measuring the femur, optimal imaging provides the most accurate measurements. Common mistakes include using an oblique plane that foreshortens the bone, not filling the entire screen with the bone, and measuring the humerus instead of the femur. When measuring the femur, it is important to keep the axis of the bone perpendicular to the probe. Measurements are obtained at the junction of cartilage and bone; the epiphysis is not included. The echogenic distal femoral point is not a true anatomic structure and, if included, results in overmeasurement of the femur (**Fig. 3**).

If the fetus is overmeasured and the fetal weight therefore overestimated, the route of delivery may be altered, namely, a cesarean delivery might be performed without a trial of labor. This route of delivery exposes both mother and fetus to unnecessary surgery and anesthesia risks (**Figs. 4** and **5**). As unfortunate as this might be, a worse scenario occurs when a fetus is undermeasured at term. In this instance, a failed attempt at a vaginal delivery could have disastrous consequences for the fetus (**Fig. 6**).

ANATOMY
Head

A common normal variant seen in the fetal head is the cavum vergae.[3] The cavum vergae, a posterior extension of the cavum septum pellucidum, could be mistaken for an abnormal cystic lesion in the fetal brain. The cavum vergae can be recognized by its characteristic location in the midline of the head, underneath (inferior to) the corpus callosum. This location can be confirmed in the sagittal plane (**Fig. 7**). The cavum vergae has no flow on color Doppler interrogation. Abnormal cystic structures such as a vein of Galen aneurysm (**Fig. 8**) or arachnoid cyst (**Fig. 9**) are recognized by their irregular margins and marked color flow in the former or by the characteristic off-center peripheral location

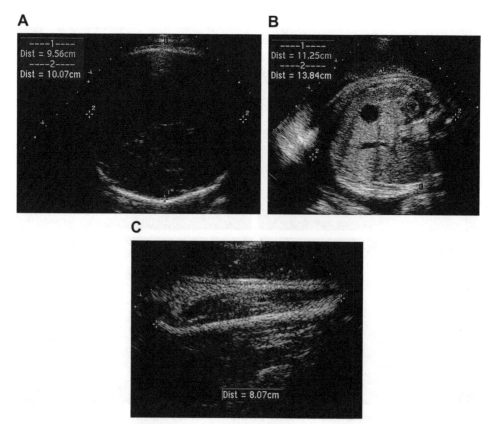

Fig. 4. Incorrect measurement technique, 40 weeks. (*A*) Short OFD, round head (BPD, 95; OFD, 101) (*B*) Overmeasured abdominal diameter (average, 123.2). Caliper 2 not on skin surface. (*C*) Overmeasured femur (81) with distal femoral point included. Estimated fetal weight using these measurements: 9 pounds, 10 ounces (96th percentile). (© M.C. Frates. All Rights Reserved.)

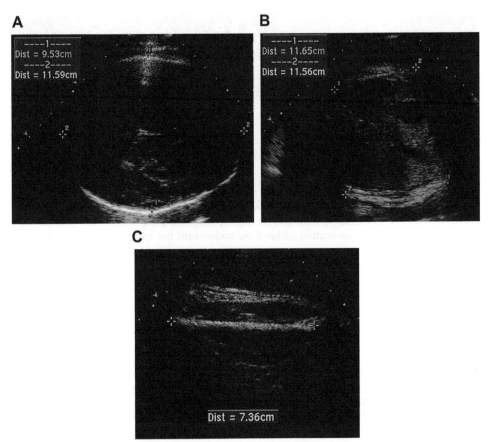

Fig. 5. Correct measurement technique, 40 weeks. Same fetus as in **Fig. 4**, with measurements obtained during the same examination: (*A*) head (BPD, 95; OFD, 116), (*B*) abdomen diameter (average, 116.5), and (*C*) femur (74) (same image as seen in **Fig. 3B**). Estimated fetal weight using these measurements: 8 pounds 5 ounces (74th percentile). Estimated fetal weight gain is half pound per week at term. Fetus was born 9 days later; birth weight was 8 pounds 11 ounces. (© M.C. Frates. All Rights Reserved.)

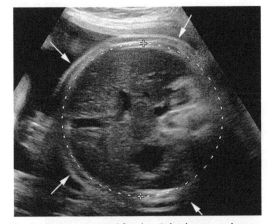

Fig. 6. Underestimated fetal weight due to undermeasurement of abdomen (subcutaneous fat excluded). Arrows point to true skin surfaces. Estimated fetal weight based on calipers on the image: 3971 g. Actual birth weight: 4859 g. Vaginal delivery was complicated by shoulder dystocia and hypoxemia; neonatal death occurred on second day of life secondary to hypoxemia and acidosis. (© M.C. Frates. All Rights Reserved.)

at the base of the brain, in the temporal lobe, or in the very high midline for the latter.

A frequent source of mistake in the assessment of the fetal head occurs when evaluating the fetus for the presence of hydrocephalus. The normal fetal lateral ventricle measures 10 mm or less at all stages of gestation.[4–7] The fetal lateral ventricle should be measured on a true axial image of the head, in the atria of the ventricle, at or just posterior to the choroid plexus.[8,9] Calipers should be placed on the inner margins of the ventricular surface and the measurement obtained perpendicular to the ventricular axis. Only the dependent ventricle can be accurately measured, but symmetry can be assumed unless there is visible evidence to the contrary. If the ventricular measurement is not obtained accurately, hydrocephalus could be incorrectly diagnosed. In the fetus with true hydrocephalus, it is impossible to obtain a normal measurement of 10 mm or less. Any error in measuring a ventricle is

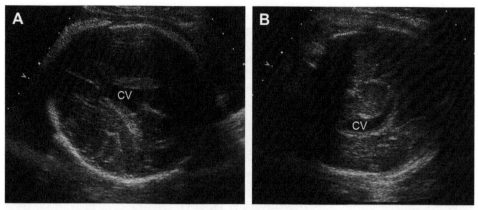

Fig. 7. Cavum vergae (CV), 33 weeks (*A*) Axial and (*B*) sagittal images of the CV. The cystic structure is located in the midline posterior to the cavum septum pellucidum, underneath the corpus callosum. (© M.C. Frates. All Rights Reserved.)

an overmeasurement because of caliper placement or an oblique image (**Fig. 10**). If multiple measurements are obtained that range from greater than to less than 10 mm, the smallest measurement is most accurate because there is no possible error that will undermeasure the ventricle. In this instance, the abnormal measurements should be disregarded and not reported as a range of the normal and abnormal measurements.

It is important to recognize one exception to the 10 mm rule for a normal lateral ventricle. In the early second trimester, the choroid plexus should fill the lateral ventricle. Early hydrocephalus can sometimes be identified by visualizing a dangling choroid, that is, the presence of a space of 3 mm or more between the medial wall of the ventricle and the medial surface of the choroid plexus. The presence of a dangling choroid raises concern for hydrocephalus, and close monitoring is required (**Fig. 11**).[10] Even in the fetus with known hydrocephalus, correct imaging is important for accurate monitoring of the intracranial process because a change in the severity of hydrocephalus in the third trimester could prompt intervention (**Fig. 12**).

Choroid plexus cysts can be identified in the fetal lateral ventricle in approximately 1% of normal pregnancies. However, this finding is also associated with trisomy 18.[11–13] A true choroid

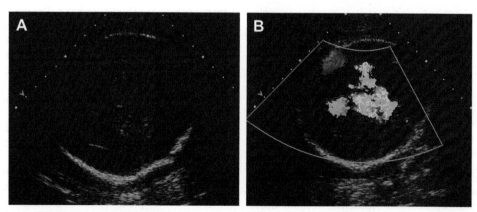

Fig. 8. Vein of Galen aneurysm, 35 weeks. (*A*) Anechoic cystic structure noted in the midline of the brain, with irregular margins. (*B*) Color Doppler interrogation shows marked vascularity. (© M.C. Frates. All Rights Reserved.)

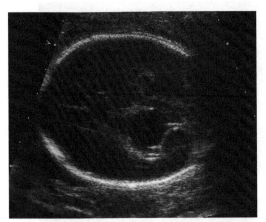

Fig. 9. Arachnoid cyst, 26 weeks. Simple cyst noted in an off-center location near the base of the brain/posterior fossa. (© M.C. Frates. All Rights Reserved.)

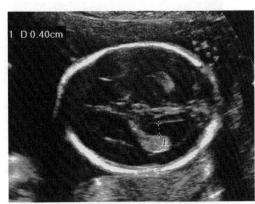

Fig. 11. Dangling choroid plexus at 18 weeks. A 4-mm gap is seen between the medial aspect of the lateral ventricle and the leading edge of the choroid. (© M.C. Frates. All Rights Reserved.)

plexus cyst is a discrete, round, anechoic structure located within the echogenic choroid. This cyst should be round in both axial and coronal planes and measure at least 2 mm in diameter (**Fig. 13**). A common mistake is to overcall a choroid plexus cyst when the lesion is an irregular or shaggy hypoechoic area in the choroid. This appearance can be termed a spongy choroid and represents a normal variant (**Fig. 14**).

The Dandy-Walker malformation sequence is characterized by absence or hypoplasia of the cerebellar vermis, with or without additional abnormalities such as hydrocephalus and cerebellar dysgenesis.[14] The normal vermis can be identified in the midline of the posterior fossa as a small round echogenic structure located between the cerebellar hemispheres and forming the posterior boundary of the fourth ventricle. An error can occur if the image of the posterior fossa is obtained in an oblique near-coronal plane rather than in the correct axial plane.[15] When imaged coronally, the vallecula of the cerebellar hemispheres can be seen projecting medially, with no intervening vermis, thus suggesting absence of the vermis (**Fig. 15**). A clue to the coronal orientation of the image is the elongation of the fourth ventricle when imaged in this plane. If the diagnosis of Dandy-Walker malformation is being considered, the imager should confirm the correct imaging plane and search for supportive findings such as flattening of the cerebellar hemispheres (**Fig. 16**). Another error

A   **B**

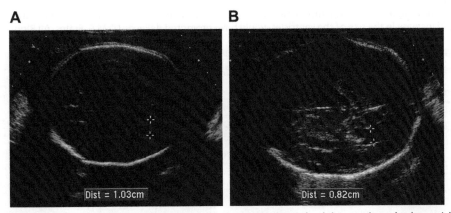

Fig. 10. Abnormal and correct lateral ventricle measurements at 30 weeks. (*A*) Lateral cerebral ventricle calipers are placed obliquely across the atrium of the lateral ventricle, thus overmeasuring the diameter at 10.3 mm. (*B*) In the same fetus, correct caliper placement perpendicular to the atrium results in a measurement of 8.2 mm. (© M.C. Frates. All Rights Reserved.)

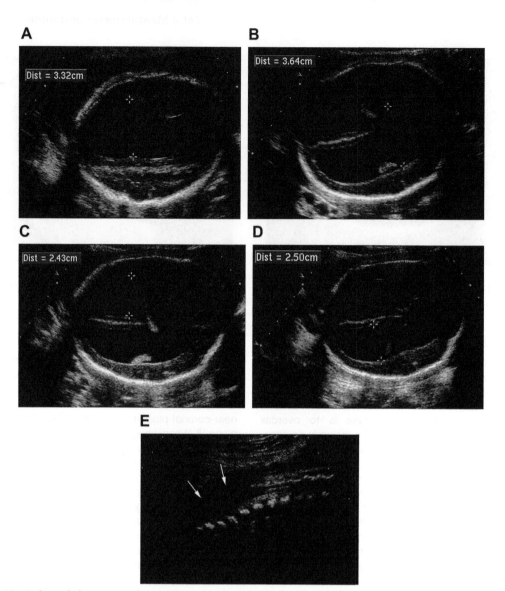

Fig. 12. Hydrocephalus measured correctly and incorrectly, 31 weeks. (*A*) Oblique measurement of the up lateral ventricle, 33 mm. (*B*) Oblique measurement of the down (dependent) ventricle, 36 mm. (*C*) Correct axial measurement of the up ventricle, 24 mm. (*D*) Correct measurement of the down ventricle, 25 mm. (*E*) Sagittal image of the lumbo-sacral spine showing a low meningomyelocele (*arrows*). Fetal ventricular size was monitored throughout the pregnancy; rapid increase in the size of the ventricles would have prompted delivery. (© M.C. Frates. All Rights Reserved.)

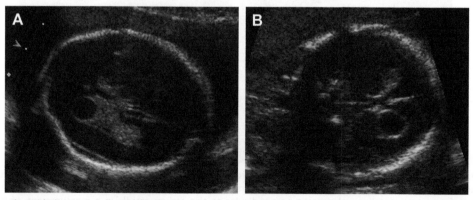

Fig. 13. Choroid plexus cyst, 19 weeks. (*A*) Axial image of the head with a discrete well-defined cyst in the posterior choroid of the dependent ventricle. (*B*) Coronal image of the same fetus; the discrete round cyst is still visible. (© M.C. Frates. All Rights Reserved.)

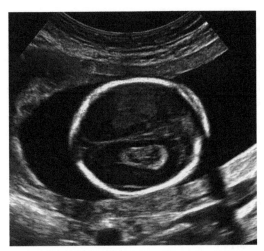

that can occur when evaluating the posterior fossa is attempting to diagnose an abnormality too early in gestation. The fetal posterior fossa does not finish developing until around 20 weeks' gestation.[16] If the fetal anatomic survey is performed earlier than 20 weeks, there is a possibility of overcalling an abnormality due to immaturity. If there is a question of incomplete formation of the vermis, repeat imaging at or after 20 weeks should be performed.

An additional posterior fossa finding that can create concern is the size of the cisterna magna. The normal size for the cisterna magna is reported to be 10 mm or less in the axial plane, with a measurement greater than 10 mm termed mega–cisterna magna (**Fig. 17**). This entity can be seen in association with other abnormalities in the fetus, particularly hypoplasia of the cerebellum and trisomy 18.[17] However, if the large cisterna magna is an isolated finding, the fetus is extremely likely to be entirely normal.[3,18] Once again, a careful search of the fetus for other abnormalities allows a reassuring report if none are found.

Face

Imaging of the fetal face is another potential source for errors. The typical face image should include the upper lip and nose, and, on this image, a prominent philtrum could be mistaken for a cleft lip (**Fig. 18**). Awareness of this issue is often sufficient to avoid overcalling a lesion. The entire upper lip and both nostrils must be visualized to exclude a cleft lip (**Fig. 19**). In addition, a normal face evaluation must include an image of both orbits (**Fig. 20**) to avoid missing the diagnosis of absence of one or both orbits, a devastating occurrence (**Fig. 21**). As with all imaging, it is much more difficult to appreciate something that is missing rather than identify something extra. Midline lesions of the face such as an anterior encephalocele may also be missed by the imager if the orbits are not

A   **B**

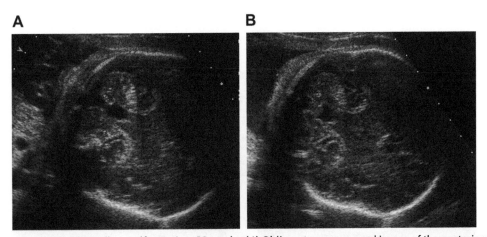

Fig. 15. Pseudo–Dandy-Walker malformation, 32 weeks. (*A*) Oblique to near-coronal image of the posterior fossa, with apparent absence of the vermis and a communication between the fourth ventricle and the cisterna magna. (*B*) Same fetus. Correct more-axial orientation of the image allows identification of the normal vermis between the cerebellar hemispheres, creating the posterior wall of the fourth ventricle. (© M.C. Frates. All Rights Reserved.)

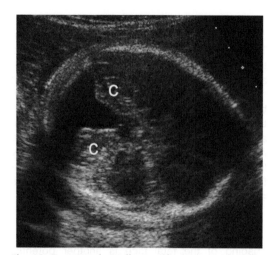

Fig. 16. True Dandy-Walker malformation, 28 weeks. Wide communication between the fourth ventricle and the cisterna magna. Note bilateral hypoplastic cerebellar hemispheres (C). Also note the axial plane of imaging. (© M.C. Frates. All Rights Reserved.)

included (**Fig. 22**). Simple cysts identified in the medial aspect of the orbits are typically dacrocystoceles, a nonworrisome process that should not be confused with pathology (**Fig. 23**). Three-dimensional imaging may provide improved imaging of the fetal face.[19,20]

Kidneys

The kidneys can be extremely subtle during the early second trimester, and the fetal adrenal glands can be quite prominent at this same gestational age. This can lead to misrepresentation of

the normal hypoechoic adrenal glands as the kidneys, which are typically isoechoic and somewhat challenging to be identified with confidence. Clues to assist in the differentiation include the more superior (cranial) location of the adrenals, often at the same level as the stomach bubble, and their typical hypoechoic triangular appearance (**Fig. 24**). The kidneys can be recognized further down in the abdomen, with occasionally a trace of fluid in the renal pelvis that, if present, confirms their identity (**Fig. 25**). A coronal color image of the abdomen to identify both renal arteries can provide useful confirmation of the presence of both kidneys (**Fig. 26**). Kidneys may be better visualized in the third trimester (**Fig. 27**).

Heart

Congenital heart disease is the most common severe congenital malformation, and imaging of the heart is technically challenging. One common pitfall in prenatal cardiac imaging that is found on the 4-chamber view is overcalling a ventricular septal defect (VSD).[21] The portion of the intraventricular septum closest to the atrioventricular (AV) valves (the membranous portion of the septum) can be very thin, and, particularly on an apical view of the heart, dropout of the sonographic beam can suggest a VSD (**Fig. 28**). When a VSD is suspected on an apical view, it must be confirmed from a different angle. In addition to the overcall of a VSD because of dropout, a VSD is commonly missed when only a static view of the heart is obtained. A videoclip of the 4-chamber view, or, better still, real time observation of the heart by a skilled examiner, is the best way to avoid missing a VSD.[22] A small VSD may not be

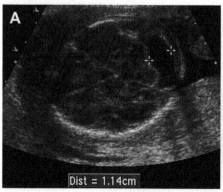
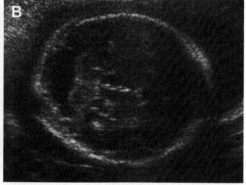

Dist = 1.14cm

Fig. 17. Mega–cisterna magna, 20 weeks. (*A*) Calipers measure an enlarged cisterna magna, 11 mm. (*B*) Same fetus, with normal-appearing cerebellum and vermis. This helps predict a good outcome despite the positive finding. (© M.C. Frates. All Rights Reserved.)

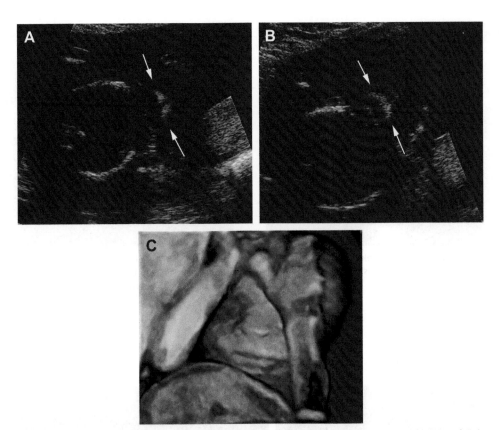

Fig. 18. Prominent philtrum mimics cleft lip, 20 weeks. (A) Oblique philtrum is seen on the superficial coronal image of the upper lip (*between arrows*). (B) Image taken slightly deeper with nose on the image showing that the upper lip is intact (*between arrows*). (C) Three-dimensional surface image confirms an intact upper lip. (© M.C. Frates. All Rights Reserved.)

visible on every 4-chamber image, and the imager should sweep through the entire septum during the evaluation of the heart. Color Doppler imaging can be very useful in the evaluation of a potential VSD. Color images should be obtained with high-velocity (scale) and low-gain settings (**Fig. 29**).

Another pitfall on the 4-chamber view is the pseudopericardial effusion.[21] This pitfall occurs

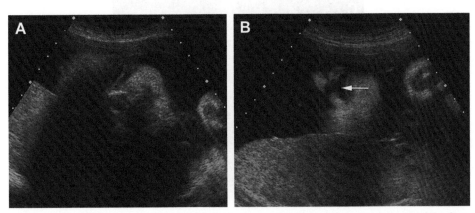

Fig. 19. Imaging plane of the lower face, correct and incorrect, 29 weeks. (A) Coronal image of the face appears normal; however, one orbit and portions of the nose and mouth are not included on the image. (B) Correct image of the upper lip and both nostrils shows a unilateral cleft lip (*arrow*). (© M.C. Frates. All Rights Reserved.)

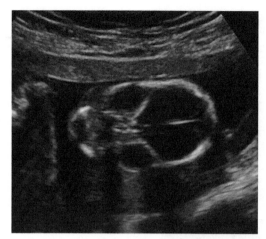

Fig. 20. Normal orbits, 20 weeks. Two distinct bony orbits are present. (© M.C. Frates. All Rights Reserved.)

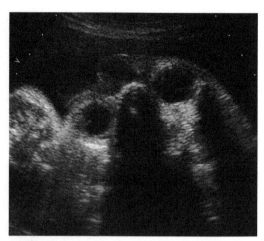

Fig. 22. Anterior encephalocele, 35 weeks. Axial image shows a soft tissue mass protruding between the orbits. (© M.C. Frates. All Rights Reserved.)

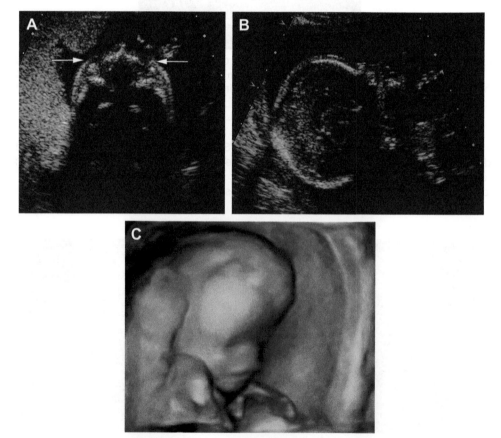

Fig. 21. Missing orbits, 21 weeks. (*A*) Axial image of the head with no orbits present (*between arrows*). (*B*) Abnormally flattened profile. (*C*) Three-dimensional surface image of flattened face with orbits missing. (© M.C. Frates. All Rights Reserved.)

A   B

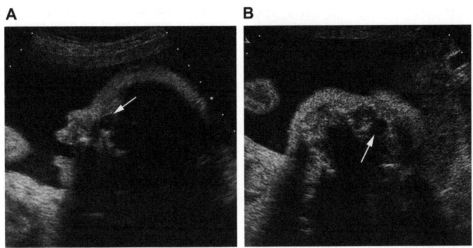

Fig. 23. Dacryocystocele, 30 weeks. (*A*) Small anechoic structure can be seen just medial to the globe adjacent to the nasal bone (*arrow*). (*B*) Axial image confirms a simple cyst (*arrow*) between the nasal bone and orbit. (© M.C. Frates. All Rights Reserved.)

when the hypoechoic external portion of the myocardium is mistaken for an effusion.[23] This mimic only extends to the level of the AV valves, whereas a true effusion extends across the level of the valves (**Fig. 30**). If a true pericardial effusion is seen, it may have no clinical significance. In the third trimester, a trace of pericardial fluid (<2 mm) is normal, and larger effusions are unlikely to indicate pathology in the absence of other cardiac abnormality.[24] The clinical circumstances of the patient (other signs of fetal hydrops, or known risk factors for hydrops such as a sacrococcygeal teratoma or tachycardia) as well as the size of the effusion assist in determining the importance of the effusion (**Fig. 31**).

Evaluation of the great vessels or outflow tracts of the heart is part of a complete fetal survey. A common mistake when evaluating the aortic

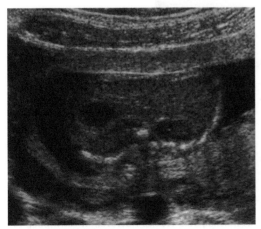

Fig. 24. Normal adrenal glands, 18 weeks. The adrenals are oval hypoechoic structures noted adjacent to the spine at the level of the stomach. (© M.C. Frates. All Rights Reserved.)

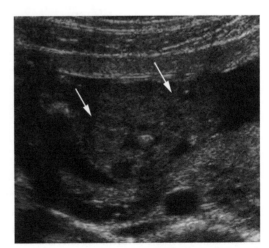

Fig. 25. Normal kidneys, 18 weeks. Same fetus as in Fig. 24. The fetal kidneys are isoechoic and subtle (*arrows*). (© M.C. Frates. All Rights Reserved.)

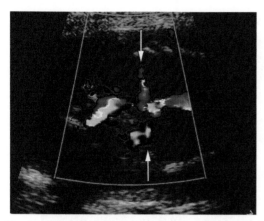

Fig. 26. Color Doppler image showing the bilateral renal arteries (*arrows*) that confirm the presence of 2 kidneys in a normal location at 19 weeks. (© M.C. Frates. All Rights Reserved.)

outflow tract is to image this great vessel in a sagittal plane. One of the most common types of congenital heart disease is tetralogy of Fallot. This malformation is diagnosed by the presence of the characteristic overriding aorta, in which the medial wall of the ascending aorta arises from the right lateral ventricle, whereas the lateral wall of the aorta arises from the left ventricle. If the aorta is only imaged in the sagittal plane, the anterior and posterior walls of the vessel are seen and the override of the medial wall is not visible. The correct plane for imaging of the aorta is just off axial, so that the intraventricular septum can be shown to be contiguous with the medial wall of the aorta (**Fig. 32**).

When imaging the fetus, careful attention to detail is critical. Being aware of common pitfalls

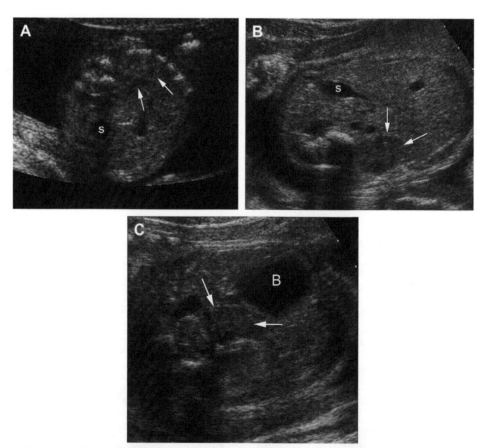

Fig. 27. Kidney anomaly overlooked. (*A*) Kidneys reported as normal, 18.5 weeks. However, in retrospect, only the right kidney is visible (*arrows*). The left renal fossa, posterior to the stomach (S), is empty. (*B*) Follow-up sonogram at 30 weeks. The right kidney is normal (*arrows*); the left kidney is absent. A small left adrenal is seen posterior to S. (*C*) Axial image of the fetal pelvis. The missing left kidney (*arrows*) is located in the midline posterior to the bladder (B). (© M.C. Frates. All Rights Reserved.)

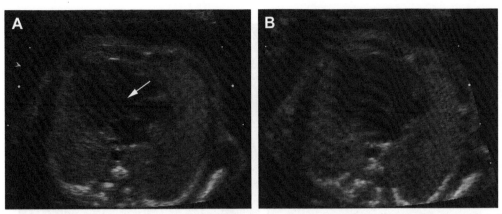

Fig. 28. Pseudo-VSD, 20 weeks. (*A*) Apical 4-chamber view shows a possible high VSD (*arrow*). (*B*) Imaging from a slightly more oblique approach confirms that the intraventricular septum is intact. (© M.C. Frates. All Rights Reserved.)

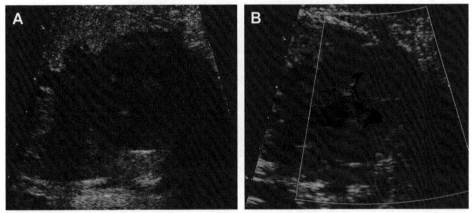

Fig. 29. Value of color Doppler in the diagnosis of a VSD, 37 weeks. (*A*) The 4-chamber view raises concern for VSD. (*B*) Adding color Doppler helps identify the high VSD, with red color indicating the flow across the septum. (© M.C. Frates. All Rights Reserved.)

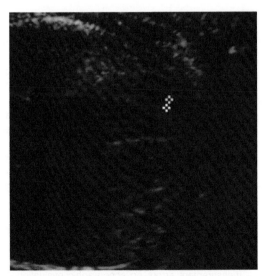

Fig. 30. Pseudopericardial effusion, 30 weeks. The hypoechoic epicardium (*calipers*) mimics a pericardial effusion; however, it does not extend beyond the level of the atrial ventricular valves. (© M.C. Frates. All Rights Reserved.)

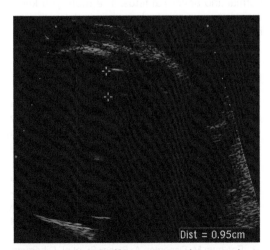

Dist = 0.95cm

Fig. 31. Pericardial effusion, 31 weeks. A moderate to large effusion (*calipers*) surrounds the entire heart. (© M.C. Frates. All Rights Reserved.)

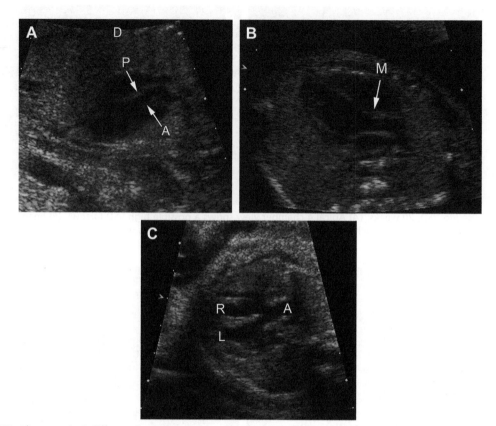

Fig. 32. The aorta in 3 different fetuses. (*A*) Unacceptable image of the aorta. The image is taken in the sagittal plane, showing the anterior (A, *arrow*) and posterior (P, *arrow*) surfaces of the vessel. Diaphragm (D). (*B*) Correct axial imaging plane. The medial wall of the aorta (M, *arrow*) is contiguous with the intraventricular septum, thus excluding an override. (*C*) Overriding aorta (A), clearly visible in the axial plane arising from both right (R) and left (L) ventricles. (© M.C. Frates. All Rights Reserved.)

can help the imager to successfully image both the normal and abnormal fetus. The more you know, the more you can look for, and, the more you look for, the more you will find.

REFERENCES

1. ACR-ACOG-AIUM practice guideline for the performance of obstetrical ultrasound. Revised 2007. Available at: http://www.acr.org/SecondaryMainMenu Categories/quality_safety/guidelines/us/us_obstetrical. aspx. Accessed August 9, 2011.
2. Galan HL, Pandipati S, Filly RA. Ultrasound evaluation of fetal biometry and normal and abnormal fetal growth. In: Callen PW, editor. Ultrasonography in obstetrics and gynecology. 5th edition. Philadelphia: WB Saunders; 2008. p. 225–65.
3. Epelman M, Daneman A, Blaser SI, et al. Differential diagnosis of intracranial cystic lesions at head US: correlation with CT and MR imaging. Radiographics 2006;26:173–96.
4. Almog B, Gamzu R, Achiron R, et al. Fetal lateral ventricular width: what should be its upper limit? J Ultrasound Med 2003;22:39–43.
5. Alagappan R, Browing PD, Laorr A, et al. Distal lateral ventricular atrium: reevaluation of normal range. Radiology 1994;194:405–8.
6. Farrell TA, Hertzberg BS, Kliewer MA, et al. Fetal lateral ventricles: reassessment of normal values for atrial diameter at US. Radiology 1994;193: 409–11.
7. Filly RA, Goldstein RB. The fetal ventricular atrium: fourth down and 10 mm to go. Radiology 1994; 193:315–7.
8. Heiserman J, Filly RA, Goldstein RB. Effect of measurement errors on sonographic evaluation of ventriculomegaly. J Ultrasound Med 1991;10:121–4.
9. Hertzberg BS, Kliewer MA, Bowie JD. Fetal cerebral ventriculomegaly: misidentification of the true medial

boundary of the ventricle at US. Radiology 1997;
205:813–6.

10. Hertzberg BS, Lile R, Foosaner ED, et al. Choroid
plexus-ventricular wall separation in fetuses with
normal-sized cerebral ventricles at sonography:
postnatal outcome. AJR Am J Roentgenol 1994;
163:405–10.

11. Ostlere SJ, Irving HC, Lilford RJ. Fetal choroid
plexus cysts: a report of 100 cases. Radiology
1990;175:753–5.

12. Naeini RM, Yoo JH, Hunter JV. Spectrum of choroid
plexus lesions in children. AJR Am J Roentgenol
2009;192:32–40.

13. Perpignano MC, Cohen HL, Klein VR, et al. Fetal
choroid plexus cysts: beware the smaller cyst. Radiology 1992;182:715–7.

14. Chang MC, Russell SA, Callen PW, et al. Sonographic detection of inferior vermian agenesis in
Dandy-Walker malformations: prognostic implications. Radiology 1994;193:765–70.

15. Laing FC, Frates MC, Brown DL, et al. Sonography
of the fetal posterior fossa: false appearance of
mega-cisterna magna and Dandy-Walker variant.
Radiology 1994;192:247–51.

16. Bromley B, Nadel AS, Pauker S, et al. Closure of the
cerebellar vermis: evaluation with second trimester
US. Radiology 1994;194:761–3.

17. Chen CP, Hung TH, Jan SW, et al. Enlarged cisterna
magna in the third trimester as a clue to fetal trisomy
18. Fetal Diagn Ther 1998;13:29–34.

18. Haimovici JA, Doubilet PM, Benson CB, et al. Clinical significance of isolated enlargement of the
cisterna magna (>10mm) on prenatal sonography.
J Ultrasound Med 1997;16:731–4.

19. Pretorius DH, House M, Nelson TR, et al. Evaluation
of normal and abnormal lips in fetuses: comparison
between three- and two-dimensional sonography.
AJR Am J Roentgenol 1995;165:1233–7.

20. Johnson DD, Pretorius DH, Budorick NE, et al.
Fetal lip and primary palate: three-dimensional
versus two-dimensional US. Radiology 2000;217:
236–9.

21. Brown DL, DiSalvo DN, Frates MC, et al. Sonography of the fetal heart: normal variants and pitfalls.
AJR Am J Roentgenol 1993;160:1251–5.

22. McGahan JP. Sonography of the fetal heart: findings
on the four-chamber view. AJR Am J Roentgenol
1991;156:547–53.

23. Brown DL, Cartier MS, Emerson DS, et al. The peripheral hypoechoic rim of the fetal heart. J Ultrasound
Med 1989;8:603–8.

24. Di Salvo DN, Brown DL, Doubilet PM, et al. Clinical
significance of isolated fetal pericardial effusion.
J Ultrasound Med 1994;13:291–3.

Gestational Trophoblastic Diseases: The Role of Ultrasound Imaging

N.J. Sebire, MD, MRCPath[a,*], Eric Jauniaux, MD, PhD, FRCOG[b]

KEYWORDS

- Hydatidiform • Mole • Choriocarcinoma
- Ultrasound • hCG

Ultrasound plays a central role in the modern management of early pregnancy complications, and is important in the identification, diagnosis, and surveillance of gestational trophoblastic disease (GTD, also known as gestational trophoblastic neoplasia (GTN). The term GTD is confusing, encompassing the range of entities in this group, such as complete hydatidiform mole (CHM), partial hydatidiform mole (PHM), invasive mole (IM), and the less common malignant choriocarcinoma (CC) and placental site trophoblastic tumor (PSTT, including a variant, epithelioid trophoblastic tumor [ETT]). The role of ultrasound in their management varies according to the specific entity, but, for the clinician, the most common and important aspect is the use of ultrasound examination for the identification of pregnancies complicated by hydatidiform mole (HM).

HM

HMs are genetically abnormal pregnancies, representing the clinical manifestation of abnormalities of imprinting of inherited genes; the differential expression according to such material is maternally or paternally inherited. The genetic abnormalities in both CHM and PHM result in absolute (CHM) or relative (PHM) overexpression of paternally derived genetic material, with resultant increased placental/trophoblastic proliferation and reduced or abnormal embryonic development. The pathognomonic feature of all molar pregnancies is therefore abnormal trophoblast hyperplasia.[1,2]

CHM are almost always diploid, with all of the genetic material being of paternal origin, usually after endoreduplication following monospermic fertilization of an anuclate oocyte or, less frequently, dispermic fertilization of an anuclate oocyte. Because the phenotype is caused by expression of only paternally derived genes, it is also possible to develop phenotypically identical CHM in an apparently genetically normal biparental diploid pregnancy in which an abnormality of genetic imprinting results in only paternal gene expression; so-called familial biparental CHM, which are at least in part caused by NALP7 maternal mutations.[3–5]

PHM also show relative overexpression of paternally derived genes, but usually caused by triploidy, with the additional set of genetic material being paternally derived. In most cases, this is caused by dispermic fertilization of an otherwise presumably normal oocyte. It is suggested that, because in PHM there is also the presence of the maternal genome, the phenotype is less severe with more prominent fetal development and less marked trophoblastic hyperplasia.[1,2]

In addition to being a specific identifiable cause of early pregnancy failure, the main clinical significance of HM pregnancy is the well-recognized

[a] Trophoblastic Disease Unit, Department of Cancer Medicine, Charing Cross Hospital, London, UK
[b] Academic Department of Obstetrics and Gynaecology, Institute for Women Health at University College London, 86–96 Chenies Mews, London, WC1E 6HX, UK
* Corresponding author.
E-mail address: SebirN@gosh.nhs.uk

Ultrasound Clin 7 (2012) 33–45
doi:10.1016/j.cult.2011.08.008
1556-858X/12/$ – see front matter © 2012 Elsevier Inc. All rights reserved.

increased risk of subsequent development of persistent GTD (pGTD), which requires treatment with chemotherapy. The risk of pGTD developing following a normal uncomplicated pregnancy is around 1 in 50,000, whereas for PHM it is around 1 in 200, and for CHM around 1 in 7.[1,2] Following identification of a molar pregnancy and evacuation of products of conception, patients should therefore undergo surveillance with blood and/or urine human chorionic gonadotropin (hCG) measurements to detect the plateauing or increasing levels associated with early pGTD development. The clinical rationale for this approach is that patients in whom pGTD is detected early have significantly less complications, and require less intensive chemotherapy, than those who present clinically with symptomatic pGTD.[6,7]

Pathology of HM

Although clinically and sonographically (see later discussion) CHM and PHM may in some cases be indistinguishable, both entities are genetically and histopathologically distinct. CHM typically shows widespread molar placental change with no appreciable fetal development, whereas PHM is associated with more advanced fetal development (although abnormal) and more focal placental hydropic change. However, histologic evidence of early embryonic development may rarely be present in cases of CHM, and most PHM are associated with early pregnancy failure in the absence of an identifiable fetus.[8–10]

The definitive diagnosis of CHM and PHM can be established using molecular genetic techniques, but such an approach is expensive and time consuming and, in routine clinical practice, the established gold standard for their diagnosis and subtyping is histopathologic examination of products of conception. With increasing experience of cases evacuated in early pregnancy, it is now recognized that CHM and PHM have distinctive histologic characteristics even in the first trimester, and their accurate diagnosis can usually be achieved based on histology alone in most cases. Molar pregnancies are histologically characterized by abnormal proliferation of villous trophoblasts, with other associated abnormalities of additional components such as blood vessels and stroma, differing between subtypes. Extravillous intermediate-type trophoblast, such as implantation site trophoblast, is important in placental site trophoblastic tumors, but is not a major diagnostic component for molar pregnancies.[8–10]

The classic textbook descriptions of both the macroscopic and microscopic features of HM are now outdated, because the introduction of modern management of pregnancy complications, including ultrasound examination, has resulted in most cases being evacuated in the late first or early second trimester. Hence, the features of marked widespread villous hydrops with extensive circumferential villous trophoblast hyperplasia and central villus cistern formation in late second trimester CHM are not usually present in most early cases. In first/early second trimester CHM, hydrops may be only minimally developed and the diagnostic histologic features are based on recognition of abnormally distributed villous trophoblast hyperplasia, sheets of pleomorphic extravillous trophoblast, collapsed villous blood vessels and marked stromal karyorrhectic debris in association with characteristic abnormal budding villous architecture and increased stromal cellularity. Extravillous trophoblast invasion is also abnormal in CHM, with a lack of the normal controlled endovascular trophoblast plugging of decidual vessels, but excessive invasive interstitial trophoblast invasion, which results in interstitial hemorrhage. Similarly, in contemporary practice, PHM shows only focal nonpolar trophoblast hyperplasia, patchy but mild villous hydrops, villous vessels containing nucleated fetal red cells, often with marked angiomatoid change, and abnormal, irregularly shaped scalloped or dentate villi, with trophoblastic pseudoinclusions and villous stromal fibrosis.[8–10]

In most cases, histopathologic features allow confident diagnosis, including all cases of CHM, but in a minority of cases the definite diagnosis of PHM may not be possible on histologic examination alone because other aneuploidies can appear histologically similar. Assessment of ploidy using in situ hybridization or flow cytometry is widely suggested to resolve this but is of limited value because of technical aspects regarding maternal contamination and, although almost all PHM are triploid, not all triploidies are PHM; digynic triploidy also results in pregnancy loss with dysmorphic villi.[11,12] Microsatellite polymorphism analysis allows definite diagnosis in all cases but is impractical for routine diagnostic practice.[13] P57[KIP2] immunohistochemistry (absent staining in CHM, positive nuclear staining in other diagnoses) allows reliable distinction between CHM and PHM, but this is usually apparent morphologically.[14,15]

Clinical Features of HM

Before the introduction of contemporary clinical obstetric and gynecologic practice, patients with HM typically presented with second trimester vaginal bleeding, uterine enlargement greater than expected for gestational age, passage of vesicles per vaginum, and associated complications such as early onset pregnancy-induced hypertension, hyperthyroidism, hyperemesis, anemia, and massive ovarian theca-lutein cysts.[16] This clinical presentation is now rarely encountered in Western countries, primarily as a consequence of the introduction of obstetric/gynecologic (OBGYN) ultrasound examination.[1,2] Pregnancies often routinely undergo first-trimester sonography for dating purposes and risk assessment for fetal abnormalities, and, even where this is not routine practice, patients presenting with first-trimester vaginal bleeding undergo routine ultrasound examination. This change in clinical care has greatly reduced the number of molar pregnancies progressing to the later second trimester, most cases now being evacuated in the late first trimester; the average gestational age at evacuation in the United Kingdom is now less than 10 weeks.[1,2] In an appropriate recent study of patients with CHM, 40% were entirely asymptomatic, molar pregnancy being detected by routine sonographic examination or following uterine evacuation, whereas the remainder presented with early vaginal bleeding; only 2% reported hyperemesis and none had any other systemic manifestations.[17]

The incidence of the different types of GTD in the first trimester of pregnancy is unknown but, because vaginal bleeding is the most common presenting symptom in most cases of CHM, the first ultrasound examination for these women is likely to take place before 12 weeks of gestation. PHMs tend to present less frequently with bleeding than CHMs (**Tables 1** and **2**) and thus the main routine clinical differential diagnosis of a molar pregnancy is a missed miscarriage of a nonmolar pregnancy.[18]

Clinical Significance

The major clinical significance of the diagnosis of CHM or PHM, apart from identifying a cause for the pregnancy loss, is the associated increased risk of development of subsequent persistent gestational trophoblastic neoplasia (pGTN), and the need for hCG surveillance.[1,2,6] Patients with pGTN, usually identified after HM based on abnormal urine or serum hCG levels, are treated with chemotherapy without a further specific histologic tissue diagnosis being made. The management of further specific complications of GTN should be performed in specialist tertiary referral centers and is outside the scope of this article.[1,2]

In cases of HM suspected sonographically (see later discussion), uterine evacuation is required as the initial management, which should be performed by suction rather than sharp curettage to minimize the risk of uterine perforation. Repeated evacuations should not be performed outside of specialist centers, because there is an increased risk of uterine perforation and, if persistent molar tissue is present, it may be deeply invasive and may require chemotherapy.[6] Ultrasound examination, both B mode and color Doppler flow assessment, has been reported to be useful to ensure completeness of uterine evacuation and identify residual trophoblastic tissue.[19,20]

Following uterine evacuation and histologic confirmation of the diagnosis, all patients should be followed up with serial hCG measurements for the early detection of pGTN.[6] In addition, once a patient has been affected by a histologically confirmed molar pregnancy, data from large registry studies have shown that there is increased risk of HM in the subsequent pregnancy; this risk is around 1% to 2% for both PHM and CHM.[21] Furthermore, because trophoblast reactivation may occur following any future pregnancy,

Table 2
Comparison of ultrasound mean gestational age (GA) at diagnosis and detection rate (DR) in CHM and PHM in retrospective studies

Author(s) (Year)	n	CHM GA (wk)	DR (%)	n	PHM GA (wk)	DR (%)
Lazarus et al,[31] 1999	21	10.5	57	—	—	—
Lindholm and Flam,[34] 1999	75	12.4	84	60	14.3	30
Benson et al,[32] 2000	24	8.7	71	—	—	—
Fowler et al,[37] 2006	253	10.0	79	606	10.0	29
Kirk et al,[38] 2007	20	—	95	41	—	20

Table 1
Comparison of the frequency of the main clinical features in CHM and PHM diagnosed during the second trimester of pregnancy

Symptoms	CHM (%)	PHM (%)
Vaginal bleeding	60	4
Uterine enlargement	25	10
Hyperemesis	10	Rare
Anemia	5	Exceptional
Multicystic ovaries	1–2	Rare
Preeclampsia	1–2	2.5

whether molar or nonmolar, hCG levels must also be checked following all subsequent pregnancies, regardless of the outcome.[6] During the follow-up period after HM, contraception is suggested because a subsequent pregnancy, and its associated hCG expression, complicates interpretation of hCG levels and hormonal effects may reactivate latent trophoblastic disease. There is controversy regarding the use of the combined oral contraceptive pill (OCP) in this setting but it seems that OCP use has no adverse effect in those women in whom there is spontaneous decrease of hCG levels to normal within 8 weeks of evacuation, whereas cases in which the hCG remains slightly increased may represent a subpopulation in whom there may be a risk of stimulating GTN growth by administered exogenous hormones. Therefore, most centers at least recommend avoidance of the OCP until hCG levels have returned to normal.[1,2]

Ultrasound in the Detection HM

Molar change within the uterus was one of the first obstetric antenatal diagnoses reported using ultrasound more than 40 years ago, with a characteristic uterine snowstorm appearance in the late second trimester.[22–24] These typical features include a uterine cavity filled with central heterogeneous mass with anechoic spaces of varying size and shape, without associated fetal development, and with bilateral large theca-lutein cysts secondary to high hCG levels producing soap-bubble or spoke-wheel appearance of the ovaries.[25,26] Because most HMs are now examined sonographically at much earlier gestations, usually secondary to vaginal bleeding, as the pathologic features are different in this setting, so are the sonographic findings. Nevertheless, several studies have reported on the use of ultrasonography for detection of HM in early pregnancy and the features of both CHM and PHM are now well recognized (**Figs. 1** and **2**).[27–39] It has been suggested that PHMs, compared with nonmolar abortions, show cystic changes and increased placental echogenicity. In a study of 21 CHM sonographically examined in both the first and second trimester (4–18 weeks) the correct pre-evacuation diagnosis of HM was made in around half the patients and no cases showed theca-lutein cysts.[31] However, similar to most sonographic diagnosis, operator experience seems to contribute to detection rates; in another study including 24 CHMs examined at a specialist center, the pre-evacuation diagnosis was made in almost 80%.[32] A further study similarly reported that, based on sonographic and macroscopic

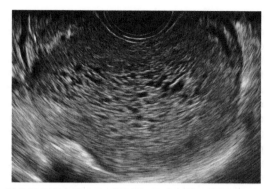

Fig. 1. A complete mole at 9 weeks of gestation. Note the complete transformation of the placental tissue giving the typical snowstorm appearance.

findings following uterine evacuation, 80% of CHMs and 30% of PHMs were identified before histologic examination.[34] Jauniaux and colleagues[33] reported that 10 of 11 pregnancies with sonographic features suggestive of HM at 10 to 14 weeks of gestation were pathologically proved to be HM, indicating that specificity of sonographic diagnosis is high, but allowing no comment on sensitivity. In these initial small studies, most cases of both PHM and CHM in which the diagnosis was not suspected before evacuation were initially sonographically reported as missed miscarriage/anembryonic pregnancy. Two larger, more recent studies have expanded these data and determined that overall, correct pre-evacuation identification of HM by ultrasound in the first and early second trimester is achieved in around 40% to 60% of cases in routine practice.[37,38] The largest study to address the issue of ultrasound findings in HM reviewed routine pre-evacuation ultrasound reports from 1053 consecutive patients referred to a UK regional

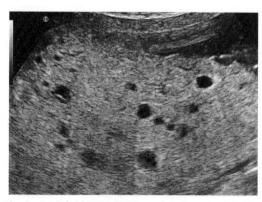

Fig. 2. A triploid PHM at 16 weeks of gestation. Note the partial transformation of the villous tissue giving the typical Swiss cheese appearance.

trophoblastic disease unit in London for histologic review of suspected HM[37]; in this setting, because all cases of possible GTN, whether suspected clinically, sonographically, or from histopathologic findings, are registered and reviewed at the center, almost complete ascertainment was possible. In this study the median gestational age at evacuation was 10 weeks (range 5–27 weeks). The final diagnosis following expert histopathologic review was HM in 859 (82%) of the referred cases, including 253 (29%) CHM and 606 (71%) PHM. Nonmolar hydropic miscarriage was diagnosed following histologic review in 194 (18%). Overall, approximately 40% of all HM cases had a correct pre-evacuation ultrasound diagnosis, including around 80% of CHMs but only 30% of PHMs (**Fig. 3**). In all sonographically unrecognized cases, the pregnancy was abnormal with the ultrasound examination detecting early pregnancy failure or missed miscarriage. In this study, which included data from a large number of referring centers, most of which were not specialist early pregnancy assessment units, there was a trend toward improved ultrasound detection rate with increasing gestational age; sonographic features of HM were reported in 35% of cases examined before 14 weeks of gestation compared with 60% examined after this time (**Fig. 4**). This study

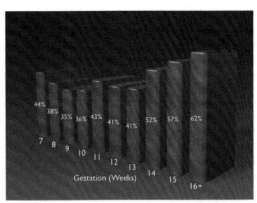

Fig. 4. Pre-evacuation detection rates of hydatidiform molar pregnancies by gestational age. There is no significant difference in detection rates across the age range but there is a trend toward improved detection rates at 14 weeks and beyond. (*Adapted from* Fowler DJ, Lindsay I, Seckl MJ, et al. Routine pre-evacuation ultrasound diagnosis of hydatidiform mole: experience of more than 1000 cases from a regional referral center. Ultrasound Obstet Gynecol 2006;27:58; with permission.)

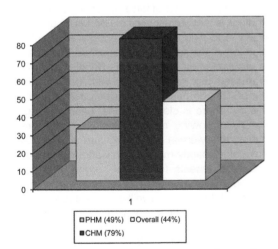

□PHM (49%) □Overall (44%)
■CHM (79%)

Fig. 3. Pre-evacuation detection rates of complete and partial hydatidiform molar pregnancies following routine sonographic examination. Less than half of all HMs (overall) in which an ultrasound examination had been performed were identified as molar before evacuation, the detection of complete moles being significantly better than for partial moles. (*Adapted from* Fowler DJ, Lindsay I, Seckl MJ, et al. Routine pre-evacuation ultrasound diagnosis of hydatidiform mole: experience of more than 1000 cases from a regional referral center. Ultrasound Obstet Gynecol 2006;27:58; with permission.)

also identified the potential false-positive sonographic diagnosis of HM in cases in nonmolar hydropic miscarriage, which represented 10% of the cases identified as HM on ultrasound examination. The sensitivity, specificity, and positive and negative predictive values for routine pre-evacuation ultrasound examination for HM therefore were 44%, 74%, 88%, and 23% respectively.[37] These data show an improvement from a similar, smaller study reporting on cases from 5 years previously, in which the overall pre-evacuation ultrasound detection rate was only 30%, suggesting improved recognition of subtle HM changes on ultrasound in early pregnancy, presumably with increasing specialization of obstetric sonographers, increasing experience in the recognition of such pregnancies, and improved ultrasound technologies.[39] Nevertheless, it is unlikely that sonographic detection rates can continue to increase much further, because of intrinsic aspects of HM at these early gestations. In a study that examined histologic features of HM in relation to whether or not they had been identified as molar sonographically, it was confirmed that those cases correctly identified had more marked hydropic villous change and that this change also increased with gestational age. However, many early, sonographically undetected cases had not yet developed significant villous hydropic change and would likely remain undetectable by routine ultrasound examination.[40]

To reliably determine the true sensitivity and specificity of ultrasound for the detection of HM in early pregnancy, in addition to examining sonographic features in histologically referred cases, it is necessary to also examine histologic findings from a patients' group selected from their sonographic findings. One study from a specialist UK early pregnancy assessment unit recruited all women suspected of having HM on ultrasound and those subsequently diagnosed with HM after histologic examination during a 4-year period. There were 56 sonographically diagnosed with HM, of whom 27 (48%) had a diagnosis of HM confirmed histologically. Overall, 61 women had HM, including 70% PHM and 30% CHM. Ultrasound findings in all cases not sonographically suspected of HM were empty sac and missed miscarriage. The overall sensitivity and positive predictive value for the ultrasound diagnosis of HM was 44% and 48%, respectively. For PHMs, the respective values were 20% and 22% and, for CHMs, 95% and 40%.[38]

Most data regarding sonographic diagnosis of HM relate to B mode ultrasound. Doppler ultrasound examination in this scenario may be additionally useful because, in the second trimester, there are usually high velocities and low resistance to flow in the uterine arterial circulation. IM appears sonographically as focal areas of increased echogenicity within the myometrium, which may appear similar to those of PSTT but occur concurrently, or soon after, a proven molar gestation. The lesion is usually heterogeneous, containing small fluid-filled cavities, and Doppler color flow mapping of the abnormal area can be used evaluate the extent of the lesion and its subsequent response to chemotherapy.[41–45] Treatment is usually with standard chemotherapy protocols or surgery, but adjunctive local ultrasound-guided injection of methotrexate has also been described.[46] In addition to initial diagnosis, ultrasonographic examination may be used as an adjunct for the detection and management of residual trophoblastic tissue within the uterine cavity.[47–52]

Clinical Implications of Sonographic Data

With current obstetric and gynecologic care, most HM present both clinically and sonographically as early pregnancy failure, with no specific features to identify them as HM. If sonographic features suggesting HM are present, it is more likely that the case represents CHM, which is the most important group to correctly identify because the risk of postmolar pGTN in this group is highest at 15%.[1,2]

Within the context of a missed miscarriage, independently of the presence of a chromosomal abnormality, the progressive changes of the villous architecture after embryonic death (before 7–8 weeks menstrual age) leads to villous hydrops, which does not herald a true PHM. Focal villous hydropic changes may also be found in pregnancies presenting with monosomy X and are probably also related to insufficient development of the villous vasculature in some placental areas as part of a larger vascular maldevelopment involving the fetal circulation or to villous degeneration in cases of placental retention following embryonic/fetal demise.[33]

However, if pre-evacuation detection of HM could become highly reliable, this would have important consequences for clinical service provision, because it would result in reduced numbers of products of conception undergoing histologic review, reduced numbers of women undergoing follow-up for equivocal histologic findings, and would allow a safe increase in the proportion of nonmolar miscarriages that could be appropriately managed medically rather than with surgical evacuation of the uterus. In the United Kingdom, Royal College of Obstetricians and Gynaecologists (RCOG) guidelines state that medical management of miscarriage is acceptable but medical methods of uterine evacuation are not recommended for suspected HM.[6,53] Because medical management of miscarriage usually results in no tissue being submitted for histologic examination, the potential danger of false-negative sonographic findings is that some cases of HM will be unrecognized and will remain unrecognized because histologic diagnosis is not possible if no tissue is available for examination. Such cases have increased risk of presenting with complications for pGTN compared with those cases identified initially. There is clear evidence, based on cases of GTN following routine terminations of pregnancy, that women presenting with clinical pGTN have significantly more complications, morbidity, and requirements for radical surgery and combination chemotherapy compared with women identified by hCG surveillance protocols.[7] It is likely that a combination of ultrasound examination and maternal serum hCG measurement using appropriate ranges for failed pregnancies would provide a significantly improved method of pre-evacuation risk assessment for GTN, but no such data regarding this combination are available. In general, molar pregnancies exhibit increased maternal hCG concentrations with associated low maternal serum α-fetoprotein concentrations. An hCG level more than 2 standard deviations more than the mean, in combination with sonography, has been suggested to identify up to 90% of cases, and, in a study of 46 HM examined at an early pregnancy assessment unit, of which 33 were suspected sonographically, in 15 cases for which hCG results were available, 9 were greater than 2 multiples of the median.[36] Further research in this area is likely to lead to significantly improved detection rates in the first trimester.

In general, there are no reliable clinical or histopathologic predictors of subsequent development of pGTN in patients presenting with HM. However, in one study of 189 patients with HM, it was reported that increased uterine size, sonographic presence of nodules, and hypervascularization on Doppler examination within the myometrium or endometrium were associated with increased risk of pGTN development.[54]

Persistent GTN

Criteria for diagnosing pGTN may differ between countries, but the principle remains that pGTN either presents with clinically apparent disease (uncommon) or on hCG surveillance (common), when it manifests as either plateauing or increasing hCG concentrations. Following the identification of pGTN, further investigations are required to stage the disease, including both uterine and liver ultrasound examination and other staging investigations according to the presentation and protocols used.[1,2] The results of these studies are used to determine the stage and prognosis score to assign patients to high-risk or low-risk groups. There are many historical staging systems for GTN, but now a more unified worldwide system has been agreed to allow comparison of outcome and treatment data across centers, the International Federation of Gynecology and Obstetrics (FIGO) 2000 (2002) Staging and Risk Factor Scoring System for GTN.[55] According to this system the criteria for the diagnosis of post-HM pGTN are: plateauing hCG for 4 measurements in a 3-week period or longer, increasing hCG on 3 consecutive weekly measurements in a period of 2 weeks or longer, histologic evidence of choriocarcinoma, and hCG level remaining increased for 6 months or more after evacuation (**Table 3**).

Imaging techniques, including ultrasound, therefore play an integral role in the initial assessment of a patient with pGTN. However, although genital tract lesions may be identified by sonography, this is most commonly in cases with high hCG levels; in those with lower hCG levels, although chemotherapy remains indicated, the uterine lesion, especially if intramyometrial, may not be visualized sonographically and, conversely, myometrial abnormalities may persist even after tumor resolution. In one series of more than 350 cases of GTN of varying types, initial sonography showed

Stage	Criteria
Stage I	Disease confined to the uterus
Stage II	GTN extends outside the uterus but is limited to the genital structures (adnexa, vagina, broad ligament)
Stage III	GTN extends to the lungs with or without genital tract involvement
Stage IV	All other metastatic sites

Table 3
International Federation of Gynecology and Obstetrics (FIGO) staging system for GTN44

molar tissue confined to the endometrial cavity in all cases of CHM, whereas, in cases of IM and CC, myometrial invasion was correctly identified.[43] Doppler studies of the uterine vasculature in HM, and in particular with pGTN and/or malignant trophoblastic tumors, usually show abnormal and significantly increased uterine blood flow with reduced flow resistance that, following evacuation, returns to normal in parallel with the serum hCG concentration, there being a correlation between hCG levels and Doppler indices throughout.[20,56–77] There are some data to suggest that uterine artery resistance may be lower at presentation in cases of GTN subsequently requiring chemotherapy, compared with those requiring uterine evacuation alone, and hence may provide additional risk stratification at presentation.[20,71,76]

Treatment of low-risk patients is with single-agent chemotherapy, usually methotrexate with folinic acid, and patients with high-risk pGTN require multidrug chemotherapy, usually based around Etoposide, Methotrexate and Dactinomycin (actinomycin-D), Cyclophosphamide and Vincristine (oncovin). The overall survival is almost 100%.[1,2] There are several publications reporting on the use of sonographic examination, usually including color Doppler assessment of uterine blood flow, for both prediction and surveillance of response to chemotherapy in pGTN, most describing similar features of GTN being associated with increased blood flow and reduced flow resistance, and there being a crude correlation between the Doppler indices and serum hCG levels. Abnormal hCG levels in association with normal uterine sonography may indicate the presence of new or residual extrauterine disease. However, although ultrasound examination, including Doppler studies, in clinical practice may provide some information regarding disease extent and response, serum hCG is a sensitive and specific marker in this context, so serum hCG levels provide the most sensitive and the simplest measure of disease extent, and this is therefore the most important clinical parameter used to monitor disease response. Occasionally, there may be residual uterine vascular malformations following pGTN treatment that may require embolization, or even hysterectomy, to control bleeding. Doppler studies may be useful to plan treatment and assess response but do not seem to predict success of embolization.[78,79]

COMPLEX DIFFERENTIAL DIAGNOSIS OF MOLAR PREGNANCIES

The coexistence of a molar placenta and apparently normal fetus often causes confusion both regarding the possible underlying pathologic basis and appropriate management. A routine antenatal ultrasound examination may show an apparently structurally normal fetus with molar change of the placenta, most often in the second or early third trimester. Several different mechanisms may result in this clinical picture and their specific features usually allow accurate antenatal diagnosis and targeted management.

PHM

Because PHM are associated with fetal development and molar placental change, it is theoretically possible that PHM may present in this way. In reality, triploid PHM usually result in early spontaneous pregnancy failure (as discussed earlier) and, when continuing into later pregnancy, the fetus almost always has structural abnormalities. The rare cases of triploidy resulting in viable delivery of a fetus probably represent mosaicism.[80] Clinically, in addition to the fetal abnormality, the placental molar changes are diffuse and patchy in nature.[33,81]

Dichorionic Twin Pregnancy with Normal Fetus and Coexisting Complete Mole

Because CHM represent abnormal conceptions, dizygotic twin pregnancies can occur with 1 otherwise typical CHM and a normal co-twin. In this setting, ultrasound examination is usually diagnostic, with an apparently structurally normal fetus with its corresponding, sonographically normal placenta, adjacent to which is a well-circumscribed and clearly delineated mass of abnormal molar placental tissue. Data from large series of such pregnancies have shown that the risk of subsequent pGTN is no greater than that reported following singleton CHM, and, furthermore, the risk of pGTN is not increased by continuing the pregnancy. However, because of the vascular and hormonal effects of the CHM, pregnancy complications are significantly increased. About half of patients develop severe vaginal bleeding with resulting spontaneous fetal loss before viability (24 weeks' gestation), and, of those who reach potential viability, 25% end in intrauterine death and 40% deliver severely preterm at less than 32 weeks' gestation. In addition, severe preeclampsia, although unusual, occurs in less than 10% of patients. Patients can therefore be counseled that the overall take-home-baby rate in those opting for continuation of pregnancy is around 30%, with a 15% to 20% chance of pGTN development and increased risk of pregnancy complications requiring intense obstetric surveillance.[82,83]

Placental Mosaicism for CHM

Mosaicism for CHM is rare, but has now been well recognized and genetically proved. Such pregnancies present with an apparently completely normal, well-grown fetus in association with diffuse molar change on ultrasound examination. The overall outcome is unknown but the best documented case resulted in live birth of a karyotypically and phenotypically normal infant with the placenta showing admixed areas of CHM and normal villi, both confirmed by microsatellite typing to be derived from the same sperm.[84,85]

Placental Mesenchymal Dysplasia

In contrast with CHM mosaicism or PHM, the most common cause of apparent sonographic diffuse cystic molar changes of the placenta in association with an apparently normal fetus is placental mesenchymal dysplasia (PMD; **Fig. 5**). PMD does not represent GTD, because there is no abnormal trophoblastic hyperplasia. There are now more than 70 well-documented cases of PMD, the

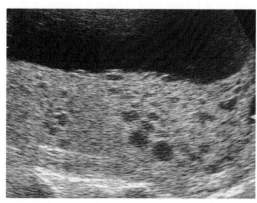

Fig. 5. A PMD at 16 weeks of gestation. Note the similar appearance of the placenta in this case with that of a PHM.

prevalence appearing to be around 1 in 4000 to 5000 pregnancies. PMD appears as diffuse molar change sonographically, with enlarged multiple cystic structures affecting the parenchyma and prominent, dilated, and tortuous chorionic vessels. Histologic findings are diagnostic, showing normal terminal villi mixed with hydropic stem villi, without trophoblast hyperplasia. In addition to the sonographic identification of cystic placental changes, maternal serum levels of hCG are increased in about 40% but, in contrast with HM, maternal serum α-fetoprotein levels are also increased in all cases in which it has been recorded. Pregnancy complications are common, including preterm delivery in 75%, intrauterine growth restriction in 20%, and intrauterine fetal death in 30%. In addition, approximately 20% of reported cases of PMD are associated with fetal Beckwith-Wiedemann syndrome and there is a marked predominance (80%) of female fetuses in association with PMD, suggesting a possible defect in imprinting. Recent data suggest that placental tissue–specific stromal compartment androgenetic-biparental mosaicism may be the underlying cause of the condition.[86–97]

Several cases of trisomy 13 presenting initially as PHM have been reported in the literature, and a recent case describes trisomy 13 presenting clinically as PHM but showing histologic changes similar to those found in mesenchymal dysplasia, further supporting the hypothesis of a primary vascular malformation of the stem villi as the main pathophysiologic basis for the changes found in the mesenchyme of the placenta in those cases.[98–100]

MALIGNANT GTD

Malignant GTD represent malignant epithelial neoplasms in which there is abnormal differentiation toward either villous-type trophoblast in the absence of chorionic villi (CC) or extravillous interstitial trophoblast (PSTT. Because all are gestational in origin, the primary site is the uterus in most cases, although, rarely, extrauterine, presumably nonmetastatic, disease can occur. By definition, such entities are malignant, so metastatic disease may occur, and distant metastases are particularly associated with CC. Malignant GTD can arise from any form of conception including CHM, PHM, normal term pregnancy, stillbirth, miscarriage, or ectopic pregnancy, but the incidence after CHM is about 1000-fold greater than following a nonmolar pregnancy.[1,2] CC following a normal term pregnancy is presumably the result of metastatic intraplacental choriocarcinoma, such primary tumors being well reported

but often microscopic so not detected sonographically or at the time of delivery.[101] CC either presents as pGTN in patients on hCG surveillance or as clinically apparent, often metastatic, disease in other recently pregnant patients, whereas PSTT and its variants often occur following a longer interval from the last known pregnancy and present with uterine symptoms such as abnormal vaginal bleeding.[1,2]

CC

Uterine CC manifests as a hemorrhagic nodule that may be in communication with the uterine cavity or may appear to be within the myometrium. Histologically, the tumor shows abnormal bilaminar villous cytotrophoblast and syncytiotrophoblastlike differentiation with coexistent marked hCG production. Viable tumor is usually seen only at the periphery of the nodule and within vascular spaces in adjacent myometrium, and the tumor does not have an intrinsic vascular supply. CC metastasizes early and secondary nodules may be present in the cervix or vagina, or distant sites, at presentation, such that any unexplained intracerebral hemorrhage or acute cor pulmonale in a woman of childbearing age should always suggest CC.[1,2] Sonographically, CC classically appears as a mass enlarging the uterus, with a heterogeneity corresponding with areas of necrosis and hemorrhage. However, there are no specific features, and CC may sonographically mimic a range of other uterine disorders.[102–106] Other imaging modalities such as computed tomography (CT) and magnetic resonance (MR) imaging are of more importance in staging and managing the disease.[1,2]

Placental Site Trophoblastic Tumor

PSTTs usually present with amenorrhea or irregular vaginal bleeding many months or even years after the last known pregnancy, and their origins from both HM and nonmolar pregnancies have been shown. The average interval from the last pregnancy is 3 to 4 years, in contrast with weeks or months for most other types of pGTN. The uterus in PSTT is usually enlarged and hCG levels are only mildly increased. Histologically, the tumor shows myometrium infiltrated by sheets and columns of intermediate-type trophoblastic cells with eosinophilic cytoplasm and nuclear pleomorphism. In contrast with CC, PSTTs usually do not metastasize early but characteristically infiltrate widely locally and may extend beyond the uterus into adjacent organs. PSTT is resistant to chemotherapy, and surgery is the treatment of choice. ETT represents a histologic subtype of PSTT.

Mortality is strongly related to the interval between presentation and the previous pregnancy.[1,2,107]

There are no specific sonographic features to reliably diagnose PSTT but, in conjunction with the history, an irregular, usually localized, uterine mass lesion may be identified. There are case reports of sonographic features of PSTT, usually showing a nonspecific mass lesion with increased vascularity, but CT and MR imaging represent the main imaging modalities once the diagnosis has been made.[108,109]

REFERENCES

1. Sebire NJ, Seckl MJ. Gestational trophoblastic disease: current management of hydatidiform mole. BMJ 2008;337:a1193.

2. Seckl MJ, Sebire NJ, Berkowitz RS. Gestational trophoblastic disease. Lancet 2010;376:717–29.

3. Wang CM, Dixon PH, Decordova S, et al. Identification of 13 novel NLRP7 mutations in 20 families with recurrent hydatidiform mole; missense mutations cluster in the leucine-rich region. J Med Genet 2009;46:569–75.

4. Messaed C, Chebaro W, Roberto RB, et al. HM Collaborative Group. NLRP7 in the spectrum of reproductive wastage: rare non-synonymous variants confer genetic susceptibility to recurrent reproductive wastage. J Med Genet 2011;48(8):540–8. PubMed PMID: 21659348.

5. Deveault C, Qian JH, Chebaro W, et al. NLRP7 mutations in women with diploid androgenetic and triploid moles: a proposed mechanism for mole formation. Hum Mol Genet 2009;18:888–97.

6. Tidy JA, Hancock BW, Newlands ES. The management of gestational trophoblastic neoplasia. Royal College of Obstetricians and Gynaecologists (RCOG) clinical guideline No. 38. London: RCOG Press; 2004.

7. Seckl MJ, Gillmore R, Foskett M, et al. Routine terminations of pregnancy–should we screen for gestational trophoblastic neoplasia? Lancet 2004;364:705–7.

8. Sebire NJ, Fisher RA, Rees HC. Histopathological diagnosis of partial and complete hydatidiform mole in the first trimester of pregnancy. Pediatr Dev Pathol 2003;6:69–77.

9. Sebire NJ, Rees H. Diagnosis of gestational trophoblastic disease in early pregnancy. Cur Diagn Pathol 2003;8:430–40.

10. Sebire NJ. Histopathological diagnosis of hydatidiform mole: contemporary features and clinical implications. Fetal Pediatr Pathol 2010;29:1–16.

11. Daniel A, Wu Z, Bennetts B, et al. Karyotype, phenotype and parental origin in 19 cases of triploidy. Prenat Diagn 2001;21:1034–48.

12. Berezowsky J, Zbieranowski I, Demers J, et al. DNA ploidy of hydatidiform moles and nonmolar conceptuses: a study using flow and tissue section image cytometry. Mod Pathol 1995;8:775–81.

13. Fisher RA, Newlands ES. Gestational trophoblastic disease. Molecular and genetic studies. J Reprod Med 1998;43:87–97.

14. Castrillon DH, Sun D, Weremowicz S, et al. Discrimination of complete hydatidiform mole from its mimics by immunohistochemistry of the paternally imprinted gene product p57KIP2. Am J Surg Pathol 2001;25:1225–30.

15. Fisher RA, Hodges MD, Rees HC, et al. The maternally transcribed gene p57(KIP2) (CDNK1C) is abnormally expressed in both androgenetic and biparental complete hydatidiform moles. Hum Mol Genet 2002;11:3267–72.

16. Santos-Ramos R, Forney JP, Schwarz BE. Sonographic findings and clinical correlations in molar pregnancy. Obstet Gynecol 1980;56:186–92.

17. Gemer O, Segal S, Kopmar A, et al. The current clinical presentation of complete molar pregnancy. Arch Gynecol Obstet 2000;264:33–4.

18. Jauniaux E. Partial moles: from postnatal to prenatal diagnosis. Placenta 1999;20:379–88.

19. Bulić M, Bistricki J, Podobnik M, et al. Evacuation of a hydatidiform mole with ultrasonic guidance. Jugosl Ginekol Opstet 1983;23:85–8.

20. Maymon R, Schneider D, Shulman A, et al. Serial color Doppler flow of uterine vasculature combined with serum beta-hCG measurements for improved monitoring of patients with gestational trophoblastic disease. A preliminary report. Gynecol Obstet Invest 1996;42:201–5.

21. Sebire NJ, Fisher RA, Foskett M, et al. Risk of recurrent hydatidiform mole and subsequent pregnancy outcome following complete or partial hydatidiform molar pregnancy. BJOG 2003;110:22–6.

22. Gottesfeld KR, Taylor ES, Thompson HE, et al. Diagnosis of hydatidiform mole by ultrasound. Obstet Gynecol 1967;30:163–71.

23. Kohorn EI, Blackwell RJ. The diagnosis of hydatidiform mole by ultrasonic B-scanning. J Obstet Gynaecol Br Commonw 1968;75(1):014–8.

24. Robinson DE, Garrett WJ, Kossoff G. The diagnosis of hydatidiform mole by ultrasound. Aust N Z J Obstet Gynaecol 1968;8:74–8.

25. Reid MH, McGahan JP, Oi R. Sonographic evaluation of hydatidiform mole and its look-alikes. AJR Am J Roentgenol 1983;140:307–11.

26. Jauniaux E. Ultrasound diagnosis and follow-up of gestational trophoblastic disease. Ultrasound Obstet Gynecol 1998;11:367–77.

27. Wagner BJ, Woodward PJ, Dickey GE. From the archives of the AFIP. Gestational trophoblastic disease: radiologic-pathologic correlation. Radiographics 1996;16:131–48.

28. Crade M, Weber PR. Appearance of molar pregnancy 9.5 weeks after conception. Use of transvaginal ultrasound for early diagnosis. J Ultrasound Med 1991;10:473–4.

29. Sherer DM, Allen T, Woods J. Transvaginal sonographic diagnosis of a hydatidiform mole occurring two weeks after curettage for an incomplete abortion. J Clin Ultrasound 1991;19:224–6.

30. Fine C, Bundy AL, Berkowitz RS, et al. Sonographic diagnosis of partial hydatidiform mole. Obstet Gynecol 1989;73:414–8.

31. Lazarus E, Hulka C, Siewert B, et al. Sonographic appearance of early complete molar pregnancies. J Ultrasound Med 1999;18:589–94.

32. Benson CB, Genest DR, Bernstein MR, et al. Sonographic appearance of first trimester complete hydatidiform moles. Ultrasound Obstet Gynecol 2000;16:188–91.

33. Jauniaux E, Nicolaides KH. Early ultrasound diagnosis and follow-up of molar pregnancies. Ultrasound Obstet Gynecol 1997;9:17–21.

34. Lindholm H, Flam F. The diagnosis of molar pregnancy by sonography and gross morphology. Acta Obstet Gynecol Scand 1999;78:6–9.

35. Woo JS, Wong LC, Hsu C, et al. Sonographic appearances of the partial hydatidiform mole. J Ultrasound Med 1983;2:261–4.

36. Johns JN, Greenwold S, Buckley E, et al. A prospective study of ultrasound screening for molar pregnancies in missed miscarriages. Ultrasound Obstet Gynecol 2005;25:493–7.

37. Fowler DJ, Lindsay I, Seckl MJ, et al. Routine pre-evacuation ultrasound diagnosis of hydatidiform mole: experience of more than 1000 cases from a regional referral center. Ultrasound Obstet Gynecol 2006;27:56–60.

38. Kirk E, Papageorghiou AT, Condous G, et al. The accuracy of first trimester ultrasound in the diagnosis of hydatidiform mole. Ultrasound Obstet Gynecol 2007;29:70–5.

39. Sebire NJ, Rees H, Paradinas F, et al. The diagnostic implications of routine ultrasound examination in histologically confirmed early molar pregnancies. Ultrasound Obstet Gynecol 2001;18:662–5.

40. Fowler DJ, Lindsay I, Seckl MJ, et al. Histomorphometric features of hydatidiform moles in early pregnancy: relationship to detectability by ultrasound examination. Ultrasound Obstet Gynecol 2007;29:76–80.

41. Taylor KJ, Schwartz PE, Kohorn EI. Gestational trophoblastic neoplasia: diagnosis with Doppler US. Radiology 1987;165:445–8.

42. Flam F. Colour flow Doppler for gestational trophoblastic neoplasia. Eur J Gynaecol Oncol 1994;15:443–8.

43. Zhou Q, Lei XY, Xie Q, et al. Sonographic and Doppler imaging in the diagnosis and treatment of gestational trophoblastic disease: a 12-year experience. J Ultrasound Med 2005;24:15–24.

44. Abd El Aal DE, El Senosy ED, Kamel MA, et al. Uterine artery Doppler blood flow in cases of hydatidiform mole and its correlation with beta-hCG. Eur J Obstet Gynecol Reprod Biol 2003;111:129–34.

45. Gungor T, Ekin M, Dumanli H, et al. Color Doppler ultrasonography in the earlier differentiation of benign mole hydatidiforms from malignant gestational trophoblastic disease. Acta Obstet Gynecol Scand 1998;77:860–2.

46. Tsukihara S, Harada T, Terakawa N. Ultrasound-guided local injection of methotrexate to treat an invasive hydatidiform mole. J Obstet Gynaecol Res 2004;30:202–4.

47. Achiron R, Goldenberg M, Lipitz S, et al. Transvaginal duplex Doppler ultrasonography in bleeding patients suspected of having residual trophoblastic tissue. Obstet Gynecol 1993;81:507–11.

48. Alcazar JL. Transvaginal ultrasonography combined with color velocity imaging and pulsed Doppler to detect residual trophoblastic tissue. Ultrasound Obstet Gynecol 1998;11:54–8.

49. Ben-Ami I, Schneider D, Maymon R, et al. Sonographic versus clinical evaluation as predictors of residual trophoblastic tissue. Hum Reprod 2005;20:1107–11.

50. Wolman I, Jaffa AJ, Pauzner D, et al. Transvaginal sonohysterography: a new aid in the diagnosis of residual trophoblastic tissue. J Clin Ultrasound 1996;24:257–61.

51. Wolman I, Hartoov J, Pauzner D, et al. Transvaginal sonohysterography for the early diagnosis of residual trophoblastic tissue. J Ultrasound Med 1997;16:257–61.

52. Zalel Y, Gamzu R, Lidor A, et al. Color Doppler imaging in the sonohysterographic diagnosis of residual trophoblastic tissue. J Clin Ultrasound 2002;30:222–5.

53. The management of early pregnancy loss. Clinical guideline no. 25 Royal College of Obstetricians and Gynaecologists (RCOG). London: RCOG Press; 2000.

54. Garavaglia E, Gentile C, Cavoretto P, et al. Ultrasound imaging after evacuation as an adjunct to beta-hCG monitoring in posthydatidiform molar gestational trophoblastic neoplasia. Am J Obstet Gynecol 2009;200:417.e1–5.

55. Benedet JL, Bender H, Jones H 3rd, et al. FIGO staging classifications and clinical practice guidelines in the management of gynecologic cancers. FIGO Committee on Gynecologic Oncology. Int J Gynaecol Obstet 2000;70:209–62.

56. Chan FY, Pun TC, Chau MT, et al. The role of Doppler sonography in assessment of malignant trophoblastic disease. Eur J Obstet Gynecol Reprod Biol 1996;68:123–8.

57. Berkowitz RS, Birnholz J, Goldstein DP, et al. Pelvic ultrasonography and the management of gestational trophoblastic disease. Gynecol Oncol 1983;15:403–12.

58. Desai RK, Desberg AL. Diagnosis of gestational trophoblastic disease: value of endovaginal color flow Doppler sonography. AJR Am J Roentgenol 1991;157:787–8.

59. Flam F, Lindholm H, Bui TH, et al. Color Doppler studies in trophoblastic tumors: a preliminary report. Ultrasound Obstet Gynecol 1991;1:349–52.

60. Long MG, Boultbee JE, Langley R, et al. Doppler assessment of the uterine circulation and the clinical behaviour of gestational trophoblastic tumours requiring chemotherapy. Br J Cancer 1992;66:883–7.

61. Murao F, Takamori H, Aoki S, et al. Ultrasonic evaluation of trophoblastic disease and the response to chemotherapy. Nippon Sanka Fujinka Gakkai Zasshi 1987;39:1137–42.

62. Long MG, Boultbee JE, Begent RH, et al. Preliminary Doppler studies on the uterine artery and myometrium in trophoblastic tumours requiring chemotherapy. Br J Obstet Gynaecol 1990;97:686–9.

63. Dobkin GR, Berkowitz RS, Goldstein DP, et al. Duplex ultrasonography for persistent gestational trophoblastic tumor. J Reprod Med 1991;36:14–6.

64. Carter J, Carlson J, Hartenbach E, et al. Persistent postmolar gestational trophoblastic disease: use of transvaginal sonography and colour flow Doppler. Aust N Z J Obstet Gynaecol 1993;33:417–9.

65. Mangili G, Spagnolo D, Valsecchi L, et al. Transvaginal ultrasonography in persistent trophoblastic tumor. Am J Obstet Gynecol 1993;169:1218–23.

66. Park YW, Kim DK, Cho JS, et al. The utilization of Doppler ultrasonography with color flow mapping in the diagnosis and evaluation of malignant trophoblastic tumors. Yonsei Med J 1994;35:329–35.

67. Hsieh FJ, Wu CC, Chen CA, et al. Correlation of uterine hemodynamics with chemotherapy response in gestational trophoblastic tumors. Obstet Gynecol 1994;83:1021–5.

68. Hsieh FJ, Wu CC, Lee CN, et al. Vascular patterns of gestational trophoblastic tumors by color Doppler ultrasound. Cancer 1994;74:2361–5.

69. Chan FY, Chau MT, Pun TC, et al. A comparison of colour Doppler sonography and the pelvic arteriogram in assessment of patients with gestational trophoblastic disease. Br J Obstet Gynaecol 1995;102:720–5.

70. Kawano M, Masuzaki H, Ishimaru T. Transvaginal color Doppler studies in gestational trophoblastic disease. Ultrasound Obstet Gynecol 1996;7:197–200.

71. Zanetta G, Lissoni A, Colombo M, et al. Detection of abnormal intrauterine vascularization by color Doppler imaging: a possible additional aid for the follow up of patients with gestational trophoblastic tumors. Ultrasound Obstet Gynecol 1996;7:32–7.

72. Bidzinski M, Lemieszczuk B, Drabik M. The assessment of value of transvaginal ultrasound for monitoring of gestational trophoblastic disease treatment. Eur J Gynaecol Oncol 1997;18:541–3.

73. Xiang Y, Yang X, Yang N, et al. A comparative study of transvaginal ultrasonography and pelvic arteriogram in assessment of patients with gestational trophoblastic tumour. Chin Med Sci J 1998;13:45–8.

74. Xie H, Hata K, Lu M, et al. Color Doppler energy and related quantitative analysis of gestational trophoblastic tumors. Int J Gynaecol Obstet 1999;65:281–6.

75. Yalcin OT, Ozalp SS, Tanir HM. Assessment of gestational trophoblastic disease by Doppler ultrasonography. Eur J Obstet Gynecol Reprod Biol 2002;103:83–7.

76. Agarwal R, Strickland S, McNeish IA, et al. Doppler ultrasonography of the uterine artery and the response to chemotherapy in patients with gestational trophoblastic tumors. Clin Cancer Res 2002;8:1142–7.

77. Oguz S, Sargin A, Aytan H, et al. Doppler study of myometrium in invasive gestational trophoblastic disease. Int J Gynecol Cancer 2004;14:972–9.

78. Lim AK, Agarwal R, Seckl MJ, et al. Embolization of bleeding residual uterine vascular malformations in patients with treated gestational trophoblastic tumors. Radiology 2002;222:640–4.

79. Ichikawa Y, Nakauchi T, Sato T, et al. Ultrasound diagnosis of uterine arteriovenous fistula associated with placental site trophoblastic tumor. Ultrasound Obstet Gynecol 2003;21:606–8.

80. Uchida IA, Freeman VC. Triploidy and chromosomes. Am J Obstet Gynecol 1985;151(1):65–9.

81. Jauniaux E, Brown R, Snijders RJ, et al. Early prenatal diagnosis of triploidy. Am J Obstet Gynecol 1997;176:550.

82. Sebire NJ, Foskett M, Paradinas FJ, et al. Outcome of twin pregnancies with complete hydatidiform mole and healthy co-twin. Lancet 2002;359:2165–6.

83. Wee L, Jauniaux E. Prenatal diagnosis and management of twin pregnancies complicated by a co-existing molar pregnancy. Prenat Diagn 2005;25:772–6.

84. Ford JH, Brown JK, Lew WY, et al. Diploid complete hydatidiform mole, mosaic for normally fertilized cells and androgenetic homozygous cells. Case report. Br J Obstet Gynaecol 1986;93(11):1181–6.

85. Makrydimas G, Sebire NJ, Thornton SE, et al. Complete hydatidiform mole and normal live birth: a novel case of confined placental mosaicism: case report. Hum Reprod 2002;17(9):2459–63.

86. Jauniaux E, Nicolaides KH, Hustin J. Perinatal features associated with placental mesenchymal dysplasia. Placenta 1997;18:701–6.

87. Moscoso G, Jauniaux E, Hustin J. Placental vascular anomaly with diffuse mesenchymal stem villous

hyperplasia. A new clinicopathological entity? Pathol Res Pract 1991;187:324–8.

88. Lage JM. Placentomegaly with massive hydrops of placental stem villi, diploid DNA content, and fetal omphaloceles: possible association with Beckwith-Wiedemann syndrome. Hum Pathol 1991;22:591–7.

89. Paradinas FJ, Sebire NJ, Fisher RA, et al. Pseudopartial moles: placental stem vessel hydrops and the association with Beckwith-Wiedemann syndrome and complete moles. Histopathology 2001;39:447–54.

90. Hillstrom MM, Brown DL, Wilkins-Haug L, et al. Sonographic appearance of placental villous hydrops associated with Beckwith-Wiedemann syndrome. J Ultrasound Med 1995;14:61–4.

91. Ohyama M, Kojyo T, Gotoda H, et al. Mesenchymal dysplasia of the placenta. Pathol Int 2000;50:759–64.

92. Matsui H, Iitsuka Y, Yamazawa K, et al. Placental mesenchymal dysplasia initially diagnosed as partial mole. Pathol Int 2003;53:810–3.

93. Cohen MC, Roper EC, Sebire NJ, et al. Placental mesenchymal dysplasia associated with fetal aneuploidy. Prenat Diagn 2005;25:187–92.

94. Kaiser-Rogers KA, McFadden DE, Livasy CA, et al. Androgenetic/biparental mosaicism causes placental mesenchymal dysplasia. J Med Genet 2006;43:187–92.

95. H'mida D, Gribaa M, Yacoubi T, et al. Placental mesenchymal dysplasia with Beckwith-Wiedemann syndrome fetus in the context of biparental and androgenic cell lines. Placenta 2008;29:454–60.

96. Reed RC, Beischel L, Schoof J, et al. Androgenetic/biparental mosaicism in an infant with hepatic mesenchymal hamartoma and placental mesenchymal dysplasia. Pediatr Dev Pathol 2008;11:377–83.

97. Hoffner L, Dunn J, Esposito N, et al. P57KIP2 immunostaining and molecular cytogenetics: combined approach aids in diagnosis of morphologically challenging cases with molar phenotype and in detecting androgenetic cell lines in mosaic/chimeric conceptions. Hum Pathol 2008;39:63–72.

98. Jauniaux E, Hadler A, Partington C. A case of partial mole associated with trisomy 13. Ultrasound Obstet Gynecol 1998;11:62–4.

99. Chen CP. Placental abnormalities and preeclampsia in trisomy 13 pregnancies. Taiwan J Obstet Gynecol 2009;48:3–8.

100. Müngen E, Dundar O, Muhcu M, et al. Placental mesenchymal dysplasia associated with trisomy 13: sonographic findings. J Clin Ultrasound 2008;36:454–6.

101. Sebire NJ, Lindsay I, Fisher RA, et al. Intraplacental choriocarcinoma: experience from a tertiary referral center and relationship with infantile choriocarcinoma. Fetal Pediatr Pathol 2005;24:21–9.

102. Sherer DM, Stimphil R, Hellmann M, et al. Transvaginal sonographic findings of isolated intramural uterine choriocarcinoma mimicking an interstitial pregnancy. J Ultrasound Med 2006;25:791–4.

103. Diouf A, Cisco ML, Lavoco A, et al. Sonographic features of gestational choriocarcinoma. J Radiol 2005;86:469–73.

104. Cormio G, Greco P, Di Vagno G, et al. Choriocarcinoma following term pregnancy by transvaginal color Doppler ultrasound. A two case report. Eur J Gynaecol Oncol 1996;17:151–3.

105. Kohorn EI, McCarthy SM, Taylor KJ. Nonmetastatic gestational trophoblastic neoplasia. Role of ultrasonography and magnetic resonance imaging. J Reprod Med 1998;43:14–20.

106. Honigl W, Reich O, Ranner G, et al. Choriocarcinoma of the uterus after term pregnancy: imaging by vaginal color Doppler ultrasound. Ultraschall Med 1997;18:165–8.

107. Schmid P, Nagai Y, Agarwal R, et al. Prognostic markers and long-term outcome of placental-site trophoblastic tumours: a retrospective observational study. Lancet 2009;374:48–55.

108. Savelli L, Pollastri P, Mabrouk M, et al. Placental site trophoblastic tumor diagnosed on transvaginal sonography. Ultrasound Obstet Gynecol 2009;34:235–6.

109. Bettencourt E, Pinto E, Abraul E, et al. Placental site trophoblastic tumour: the value of transvaginal colour and pulsed Doppler sonography (TV-CDS) in its diagnosis: case report. Eur J Gynaecol Oncol 1997;18:461–4.

The Role of Ultrasound in the Management of Threatened Miscarriage

Michelle Swer, BSc, MBBS, MRCOG,
Davor Jurkovic, MD, FRCOG, Eric Jauniaux, MD, PhD, FRCOG*

KEYWORDS
- Bleeding • Hematoma • Miscarriage • Pregnancy
- First trimester • Obstetric outcome

Placental-related disorders of pregnancy are the most common complications of human pregnancies. Collectively, complete missed miscarriages, recurrent miscarriages and threatened miscarriage (TM), and placental insufficiency associated or not with maternal hypertensive disorders affect more than 30% of clinical pregnancies in humans. These placental disorders are exceptional in other mammalian species.[1,2]

First-trimester vaginal bleeding is the most common symptom of complications during pregnancy, occurring in 14% to 20% of women.[2–5] TM is diagnosed when a normally grown live fetus of less than 24 weeks is found on ultrasound in the presence of vaginal bleeding.[3–6] The causes of vaginal bleeding are separated into intrauterine causes and extrauterine causes (including the cervix). Intrauterine causes of bleeding are almost always caused by the breakdown of 1 or more uteroplacental vessels connecting the maternal circulation with the placental intervillous room. Bleeding from umbilicoplacental vessels is exceptional and the blood is usually contained between the amniotic membrane and fetal plate of the placenta.[6] The resulting subamniotic hematomas are sometimes mistaken on ultrasound for subchorionic hematomas.[7]

The prevalence of TM with or without a visible intrauterine hematoma (IUH) is a constant throughout the world. Most TMs occur during the first trimester and the outcome of pregnancy is influenced by the gestational age at the onset of symptoms.[2–5] TM is associated with focal oxidative stress in the definitive placenta, which increases the risk of adverse pregnancy outcomes such as miscarriage, preterm delivery, and premature rupture of the membranes. It has been reported that 2% to 12% of women[2–5] who initially present with TM eventually suffer a complete miscarriage. The risk is higher in early pregnancy and tends to decrease once the presence of embryonic cardiac activity has been confirmed.[3,4] Little is known about the short-term and long-term consequences of these complications and subsequent ongoing pregnancies. Most available data come from small retrospective series. Large series describing specific complications have been published, but there are inconsistencies in the terminology and the definitions that were used to describe adverse outcomes.[2]

Various management protocols have been developed, including conservative management and hormonal therapy based on progesterone and human chorionic gonadotrophin (hCG). TM

Academic Department of Obstetrics and Gynaecology, Institute for Women Health at University College London, 86–96 Chenies Mews, London, WC1E 6HX, UK
* Corresponding author.
E-mail address: e.jauniaux@ucl.ac.uk

Ultrasound Clin 7 (2012) 47–55
doi:10.1016/j.cult.2011.08.007

often causes anxiety to women because bleeding in early pregnancy can lead to pregnancy loss and other obstetric complications. This article evaluates the available clinical evidence on the pathophysiology and epidemiology of TMs and the clinical diagnosis and management of women presenting with bleeding of an intrauterine origin in early pregnancy.

PATHOPHYSIOLOGY

Intrauterine bleeding during early pregnancy most often originates from the uteroplacental circulation between the forming chorionic membrane and the uterine wall.[2–5] Depending on the location of the bleed, this can result in the formation of an IUH. The formation of a subchorionic (SC) IUH (**Fig. 1**) between the placental villous tissue or membranes and the uterine wall may disrupt placentation. If the hematoma expands to the rest of the placental mass, it will dislocate and disrupt the maternoplacenta interface and result in full miscarriage if the damage expands rapidly to the definitive placental tissue. In the long term, bleeding in the periphery of the definitive placenta or in the free membranes can lead to partial or complete detachment of the placenta (placental abruption), preterm premature rupture of fetal membranes (PPROM), low birth weight (LBW), persistent gestational trophoblastic disease (PGTD), premature delivery (PTD) and intrauterine death (IUD).[2–5,8–11] The pathophysiology of these complications is linked to chronic oxidative stress within the decidua and/or the free membranes, resulting in focal weakening and rupture of the membranes and/or resulting in premature myometrial activity.[1]

There is increasing evidence that failures of placentation are associated with an imbalance of free radicals, which further affects placental development and function and may subsequently have an influence on both the fetus and the mother.[1,12,13] The placental syncytiotrophoblast is extremely sensitive to oxidative stress, partly because it is the outermost tissue of the conceptus and so exposed to the highest concentrations of oxygen coming from the mother, and partly because it contains low concentrations of the principal antioxidant enzymes, particularly in early pregnancy.

Human placentation is characterized by the highly invasive nature of the conceptus, which embeds itself completely within the maternal uterine endometrium and superficial myometrium and by a remodeling of the tip of the maternal spiral arteries.[1] In normal pregnancies, the earliest stages of development take place in a low-oxygen (O_2) environment.[1,12,13] This physiologic hypoxia of the early gestational sac protects the developing fetus from the deleterious and teratogenic effects of O_2 free radicals. A stable O_2 gradient between the maternal uterine decidua and the fetoplacental tissue is also an important factor in trophoblast differentiation and migration, normal villous development, and angiogenesis.[14,15] Our previous studies have shown that, in normal pregnancies, there is a physiologic oxidative stress in the placental tissue at around 9 to 10 weeks that is shown by an increase in HSP70 activity, mainly in the periphery of the primitive placenta.[16,17] The villous changes observed in the periphery of the placenta during the formation of the fetal membranes are identical to those found in the missed miscarriage (early embryonic demise), indicating a common mechanism mediated by oxidative stress.[18,19] These changes cannot be observed retrospectively in pregnancies that continue after a first-trimester bleed; however, IUHs can persist for several weeks on ultrasound, suggesting that a focal excessive stress in the definite membranes can lead to a chronic inflammatory reaction within the decidua and membranes. If bleeding is limited or happens close to the internal cervical os and is evacuated, the pregnancy may continue and the inflammatory reaction will trigger most of the obstetric complications observed after first-trimester TM.

EPIDEMIOLOGY AND OBSTETRIC OUTCOME

An association between TM and subsequent adverse obstetric outcomes has been studied for decades. However, most studies are small, retrospective, and noncontrolled, which limits their value. A few systematic reviews and meta-analysis are now available.[9–11]

Vaginal bleeding before 24 weeks has been shown to be associated with an increased risk of

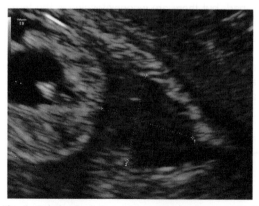

Fig. 1. Subchorionic hematoma developing next to 6 weeks' gestational sac.

subsequent placental/membrane-related obstetrics complications and these risks seem to be higher in women presenting with heavy and chronic bleeding during the first half of pregnancy (**Table 1**). TM is associated with a twofold increased risk of antepartum hemorraghe in the second and third trimester and placental abruption.[9,10] The risk of placenta previa also seems to be increased after TM but the position of the placenta in early pregnancy is likely to be the cause of the bleeding rather than the consequence. Fetuses of women presenting with heavy bleeding are at higher risk of being small for gestational age (SGA), whereas those with light bleeding are not at increased risk (the risk of SGA increases with the heaviness of vaginal bleeding).[9] In almost all studies, a 1.9-fold to 3.7-fold increased risk of PPROM has been observed as well as an increased risk of PTD, in particular after heavy bleeding.[9–11] As a consequence, the mean birthweight after TM has been found to be lower than in controls.[9] Other abnormal perinatal outcomes, including pregnancy-induced hypertension (PIH), low 5-minute Apgar score, IUD, and perinatal deaths seem to be unaffected after TM, but the risk of congenital malformation seems to be increased.[2] A recent small study showed that the combination of bleeding in early pregnancy and advanced age increases risk of pregnancy loss even after ultrasound has confirmed fetal heart activity.[20] However, the risk of miscarriage is directly linked to maternal age, so this finding is probably only coincidental. Previous studies have shown that vaginal bleeding in very early pregnancy (ie, before 6 weeks of gestation) does not seem to be associated with any immediate or long-term consequences.[21]

The risk of subsequent miscarriage is independent of presence/absence of vaginal bleeding and the size and the localization of the Subchorionic intra-uterine hematoma (SCIUH).[4,5] The risk of miscarriage is 2.4-fold higher when the SCIUH is diagnosed between 7 and 9 weeks' gestation.[22,23] The presence of an SCIUH is associated with an increased risk for PIH, preeclampsia (PE), placental abruption, PTD, SGA, fetal distress, and SCIUH (see **Table 1**). The risk of PTD seems to be independent of the presence or absence of vaginal bleeding. There are no data on the risk of LBW or very low birth weight (VLBW) but the risk of congenital anomalies and perinatal death seems not to be increased in cases of an SCIUH. A recent systematic review and meta-analysis on the perinatal outcomes of women presenting with an SCIUH found 7 studies including 1735 women with subchorionic hematoma and 70,703 controls who met inclusion criteria.[11] An SCIUH was associated with an increased risk of miscarriage (from

Table 1
Obstetric outcome following TM with mild and heavy per-vaginal bleeding (PVB), the presence of an IUH

Obstetric Outcome	Mild PVB	N	Heavy PVB	N	IUH	N
Hemorrhage	1.8 (1.7–1.9)	2	No data	0	No data	0
PIH	1.4 (1.1–1.8)	1	1.1 (0.5–2.4)	1	2.1 (1.5–2.9)	1
PE	1.2 (0.9–1.6)	2	1.1 (0.5–2.4)	1	4.0 (2.3–7.0)	1
Placental abruption	1.8 (1.1–2.9)	3	3.6 (1.6–7.9)	1	6.4 (3.4–12.2)	2
Placenta previa	1.5 (0.8–2.9)	3	2.5 (0.9–6.9)	1	No data	0
PPROM	1.3 (1.0–1.7)	3	3.2 (1.8–5.7)	1	0.7 (0.1–3.2)	1
PTD<37 wk	1.6 (1.4–1.8)	8	2.4 (1.0–5.8)	3	2.4 (1.7–3.3)	4
PTD<34 wk	2.5 (1.6–3.9)	4	No data	0	No data	0
IUGR	No data	0	No data	0	No data	0
SGA	1.4 (1.0–1.9)	2	2.6 (1.2–5.6)	1	2.1 (1.4–3.3)	3
LBW<2500 g	1.6 (1.1–2.2)	5	1.7 (0.9–3.3)	1	No data	0
LBW<1500 g	2.7 (1.4–5.2)	3	No data	0	No data	0
Fetal death	1.1 (0.8–1.4)	4	No data	0	2.8 (0.9–8.4)	2
Perinatal death	2.1 (1.0–4.4)	4	No data	0	2.1 (0.8–5.4)	2

Data are reported as the odds ratio with 95% confidence interval.

Abbreviations: IUGR, in utero growth retardation; LBW, low birth weight; N, number of studies; PE, preeclampsia; PIH, pregnancy-induced hypertension; PTD, persistent trophoblastic disease; PVB, per-vaginal bleeding; SGA, small for gestational age.

Modified from van Oppenraaij RH, Jauniaux E, Christiansen OB, et al. Predicting adverse obstetric outcome after early pregnancy events and complications: a review. Hum Reprod Update 2009;15:409–21.

8.9% to 17.6%) and stillbirth (from 0.9% to 1.9%). The number needed to harm was 11 for miscarriage and 103 for stillbirth, meaning that 1 extra miscarriage is estimated to occur for every 11 women with SCIUH diagnosed, and 1 extra stillbirth occurs for every 103 women with SCIUH diagnosed. Women with an SCIUH are also at increased risk of abruption (from 0.7% to 3.6%), preterm delivery (from 10.1% to 13.6%), and preterm premature rupture of membranes (from 2.3% to 3.8%).

CLINICAL EVALUATION
The Role of Ultrasound

Ultrasound is essential for the differential diagnosis between a TM, a missed miscarriage, an incomplete miscarriage, and an extrauterine pregnancy. There are several morphologic features that can be assessed to estimate the likelihood of favorable pregnancy outcome, especially in women with a TM.

The shape, position, and trophoblastic reaction of the gestation sac can be predictive of early pregnancy failure.[24] A sac with an irregular or angular appearance is associated with an increased risk of miscarriage. The low position of the gestation sac within the uterine cavity and the finding of a thin trophoblast shell are additional subjective findings that denote a poor prognosis.

In a normal early pregnancy, the size of the gestation sac may be used to estimate gestational age. The sac appears between 4.5 and 5 weeks' gestation and grows approximately 1 mm per day during the first trimester. An embryo can be seen within a gestation sac, which is as small as 10 mm.[25] A gestational sac of more than 20 mm in diameter with the absence of an embryo is an indicator of early embryonic demise (**Fig. 2**). However, there is considerable variability in determining the optimal cutoff for the size of the

gestation sac in establishing a miscarriage. Different studies have shown cutoff points of 16 mm, 17 mm, or 18 mm as possible predictors for nonviability.[24–26] However, Elson and colleagues[27] showed that normal pregnancies may occasionally present with a gestation sac greater than 18 mm with no visible embryo on the initial scan.

Abnormal developmental pattern of fetal heart rhythm (FHR) and/or bradycardia has been associated with subsequent miscarriage. In particular, a slow FHR at 6 to 8 weeks seems to be associated with subsequent fetal demise.[7] A single observation of an abnormally slow heart rate does not necessarily indicate subsequent embryonic death, but a continuous decline of embryonic heart activity is inevitably associated with miscarriage.

SCIUHs are defined on ultrasound as crescent-shaped echolucent areas between the chorionic membranes and/or placenta and the myometrium.[4,5] An understanding of the resolution of these hematomas and the prognostic relevance of this ultrasound finding is limited because much emphasis has been put on the volume of an SCIUH or on the presence of vaginal bleeding but not on the location of the bleed.[23,28–32] Recent hematomas are hyperechogenic to isoechogenic compared with the placenta, whereas resolving hematomas become hypoechogenic within 1 week and sonolucent within 2 weeks. An SCIUH is found on ultrasound in 18% to 39% of the women presenting with TM, and around 70% of women diagnosed with an IUH on ultrasound experience vaginal bleeding. If the bleeding occurs at the level of the definitive placenta (under the cord insertion), it is likely that it will result in placental separation and subsequent miscarriage. Conversely, an SCIUH only detaching the membrane opposite to the cord insertion can probably reach a significant volume before it affects normal placental and fetal development. Subchorionic bleeding can affect pregnancy outcome in several ways. In theory, a large hematoma can pose a threat to the continuance of the pregnancy by a direct volume-pressure effect and, in the second trimester, must differentiate from a large placental lake that is within the placental tissue and contains slow turbulent maternal blood flow (**Fig. 3**). This differentiation may depend on the site of the hematoma, its distance from the site of the placenta, and the volume of the hematoma. Ultrasound has proved to be useful in aiding with prognostic factors regarding the outcome of TM. However, these findings are not specific enough to make a conclusive diagnosis and further scans are usually necessary to monitor the progress of pregnancy.

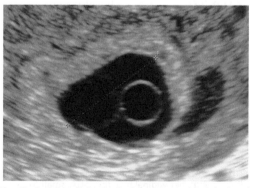

Fig. 2. Small subchorionic hematoma (*right*) developing next to a 7 weeks' gestational sac containing only a dilated secondary yolk sac.

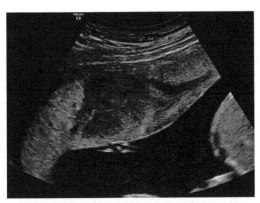

Fig. 3. Large intraplacental lake at 18 weeks of gestation containing turbulent slow maternal blood. The lake is an area of no placental tissue between 2 cotyledons.

The Role of Maternal Serum Biology

In early pregnancy failure, the development of the placentodecidual interface is severely impaired, leading to early and widespread onset of maternal blood flowing continuously inside the placenta, together with major oxidative stress–induced tissue degeneration. This oxidative stress and increase in oxygenation associated with placental malfunction has an impact on the synthesis of various placental proteins. Many studies have investigated whether these proteins can be used as predictors of early pregnancy loss, with varying success.

Maternal serum hCG and progesterone are the most commonly used markers in the assessment of pregnancy viability. Both serum markers play a vital role in the maintenance of pregnancy viability. There have been extensive studies of their patterns and secretions in both normal and failing pregnancies. Lower levels of maternal serum hCG (MShCG) and progesterone in pregnancies that are destined to fail have been well documented. A single MShCG measurement has a sensitivity of 88% in distinguishing between viable and nonviable pregnancies.[33] Some studies have used serial measurements of hCG as a means of predicting outcome,[34] although this requires several days of monitoring, which is not useful when applied in a clinical setting. A more recent study has evaluated a combination of MShCG and progesterone in predicting the outcome of TM and found sensitivity of 88.1% and specificity of 84.3%.[35]

Investigations have also been performed on other serum markers such as pregnancy-associated plasma protein A (PAPP-A) and inhibin-A. PAPP-A is used routinely in the first and second trimester screening of Down syndrome. However, it has been found to be low in the first trimester in association with miscarriage, but studies have found it to be of low predictive value for fetal demise.[36] Inhibin-A has also been shown to have autocrine and paracrine effects on placental hormone production. These serum markers, in combination with hCG, have been shown to be useful in predicting those pregnancies presenting with TM that are destined to fail. A previous study of a combination of hCG, progesterone, PAPP-A, and inhibin-A showed decreased levels in the first trimester in patients with symptoms of TM, with a logistic regression analysis highlighting inhibin-A as the best predictor of subsequent full miscarriage.[37]

More recently studies have evaluated the role of angiogenic factors and cytokines in early pregnancy complications. Angiogenesis is characterized by increased vascular permeability and endothelial cell proliferation and migration, which is regulated by various proangiogenic and antiangiogenic factors, angiopoietins, and matrix metalloproteinases. In recent years proangiogenic and antiangiogenic proteins have been reported to be useful biomarkers in predicting pregnancy complications such as preeclampsia and fetal growth restriction. A recent study compared levels of maternal serum levels of angiogenic factors soluble vascular endothelial growth factor (VEGF) receptor 1 (sFLT-1), placental growth factor (PlGF), and soluble endoglin in women with symptoms of TM compared with asymptomatic controls and nonpregnant women in the luteal phase. The results showed that maternal SFLT-1 and PlGF were distinctly lower in TM complicated by subsequent miscarriage (83% and 44% decrease respectively) compared with normal pregnant controls and TM with subsequent live birth.[38] The numbers in the study were small but they show that, with further research on larger sample sizes, these are potential sensitive predictors of a subsequent miscarriage in patients with TM in the first trimester.

Cytokines are known to play an important role in implantation, with a strong association existing between maternal T helper-1 (Th1)–type immunity and pregnancy loss, thus causing an imbalance in cytokine (Th1/Th2) production. This increased Th1 type of immune response is documented in women with recurrent or complete miscarriage.[39] Proinflammatory cytokine receptors such as tumor necrosis factor α (TNFα) have been associated with threatened abortions.[40] They have also been associated with preterm deliveries[41] and have been used in first-trimester screening for patients at risk of preeclampsia.[42] A recent study evaluated these changes in levels of cytokines and the role they could play in the prediction of risk of miscarriage in women with a TM.[43] The study shows that monocyte expression of TNFα and circulating levels of TNFα, interferon γ (IFNγ), interleukin (IL)-10, IL-6, and TNF-R1 were significantly lower, whereas circulating levels of TNFα/IL-10, IFNγ/IL-10, and TNFα/IL-6 ratios were significantly higher, in women with TM who subsequently miscarried, compared with the women with normal outcome. These findings are similar to those from women with recurrent or complete miscarriage. The immune response is also similar to that seen in preterm labor, as mentioned earlier. The study suggests the possibility of cytokines being used in combination with other biomarkers as predictors of early pregnancy outcome in a clinical setting.

The role of serum biology in the prediction of outcome of pregnancy in women with TM is still novel, largely because of the small numbers in most of the studies. However, the results have shown a strong association of these molecules as possible predictive markers, which needs further analysis before they can be used clinically.

MANAGEMENT

Several interventions have been used for preventing a poor outcome following bleeding in early pregnancy. Attempts to maintain the pregnancy are likely to be more successful if a viable fetus is identified on ultrasound and if the risk of a chromosomal abnormality is low (ie, in younger women).

Bed Rest

Bed rest is a commonly used management practice in antenatal care, with up to 95% of obstetricians advising it for some complication in their practice.[44] The first study was performed in 1953[45] and found that normal physical activity was no more likely to lead to a poor outcome in TM than bed rest; however, bed rest was advised in these cases to control maternal blood loss. This advice has continued to be given to women at risk of miscarriage or with a history of recurrent miscarriages.

More recent studies have evaluated the effectiveness of bed rest in early pregnancy. A prospective observational study in 2003 of all women with a TM complicated by a subchorionic hematoma who were advised bed rest compared outcomes between those who were compliant (n = 200) and those who were not (n = 30). The results showed a miscarriage rate of 9.9% in those who took bed rest compared with 23.3% in those who carried on with their daily activities.[46] However, the 2 groups had an uneven balance in numbers

that may bias the findings. A Cochrane review of randomized controlled trials (RCTs) compared clinical outcomes in pregnant women who were prescribed bed rest at home or in hospital compared with alternative care or no intervention. Two trials were identified that studied bed rest as an intervention.[47,48] Neither trial showed any significance in an increased risk of miscarriage in the bed rest group compared with the other groups, although the sample sizes were small.

The most likely cause of a miscarriage is fetal or congenital anomalies and, therefore, the restriction of physical activity is unlikely to have any direct impact on the outcome of a TM. As advised by the Cochrane review, future RCTs need to be performed on larger numbers and other factors, such as the risk of thromboembolic events, women's satisfaction, psychological adjustment, and cost implications.[49] Although it is still used frequently, bed rest is not recommended as a routine management.

Hormonotherapy

The physiologic roles of both progesterone and hCG in the establishment and maintenance of pregnancy has led to their use as therapeutic agents in TM with the aim of preserving the pregnancy.

Low secretory levels of progesterone have been linked to miscarriage. Hence supplementation of progesterone has been used in women with TM or presumed progesterone deficiency to help maintain the pregnancy. There have been several studies of the efficacy of progesterone as a therapeutic agent. However, a recent Cochrane review described most of these studies as being of poor methodological quality.[50] Only 2 studies were included in the review. Both studies randomized patients to treatment versus placebo and evaluated outcomes of miscarriage and preterm labor,[51] and pain and uterine contractions.[52] A meta-analysis of the effects of the progesterone on miscarriage compared with placebo showed a reduction of miscarriage rate with the use of progesterone (relative risks [RR] 0.47, 95% confidence interval 0.17–1.3).[50] However, the sample size was small and the method of randomization was unclear in both trials, making them methodologically poor. Hence, the evidence to support the routine use of progesterone in the management of TM is still uncertain.

Similar results are seen with the use of hCG as treatment of TM. Like progesterone, there has been a lot of interest in the effectiveness of hCG as a treatment regimen. A meta-analysis of studies performed by the Cochrane review showed no statistical significance on the effect of miscarriage (RR 0.83; 95% confidence interval 0.46–1.47) when comparing treatment with placebo.[53] There was a significant reduction in the risk of miscarriage when comparing the use of hCG with bed rest, but it was thought that 1 of the trials was of poor methodological quality and that this influenced the results. Overall, the available data are not sufficient to support the routine use of hCG in treating TM.

Other Regimens

Increased uterine activity has been associated with TM, although it is unclear whether it arises from a cause or effect. However, this association has led to the possibility of the use of drugs such as antispasmodics and tocolytic agents if they can reduce uterine activity and thus continue the pregnancy.

The use of these drugs is popular in South America, although there is little evidence of studies performed on them. Most of the studies performed on uterine muscle relaxants were conducted more than 20 years ago. One RCT compared buphenine with placebo and found a lower risk of miscarriage associated with the use of the β-agonist compared with the placebo.[54] However, the methodological quality of this study is unclear. Not enough work has been done on these drugs to use them routinely in TM.

Overall, the various treatment options used in the management of TM have little evidence to support them as routine policies. Ultrasound scans, usually 10 days to 2 weeks after a diagnosis of TM, are advised to confirm the outcome.[55]

SUMMARY

TM is associated with an increased risk of adverse obstetric and perinatal outcomes, including higher risk of LBW and VLBW after a simple TM episode and higher risk of PIH, PE, placental abruption, PTD, SGA, and low 5-minute Apgar score after the detection of an SCIUH. Ultrasound enables a conclusive diagnosis in most normal pregnancies and early pregnancy abnormalities. However, maternal serum biochemistry can be useful in helping to predict early pregnancy outcomes in cases that are not straightforward. Ultrasound findings and maternal serum biochemistry, together with the clinical history, provide valuable information about the prognosis of TM and are important to determine potential management options. More studies on these common early pregnancy complications should enable better management protocols and new therapeutic guidelines to improve the perinatal outcome in women at higher risk of abnormal pregnancy outcome.

REFERENCES

1. Jauniaux E, Poston L, Burton GJ. Placental-related diseases of pregnancy: involvement of oxidative stress and implications in human evolution. Hum Reprod Update 2006;12:747–55.
2. Jauniaux E, Van Oppenraaij RH, Burton GJ. Obstetric outcome after early placental complications. Curr Opin Obstet Gynecol 2010;22:452–7.
3. Johns J, Hyett J, Jauniaux E. Obstetric outcome after threatened miscarriage with and without a hematoma on ultrasound. Obstet Gynecol 2003; 102:483–7.
4. Johns J, Jauniaux E. Threatened miscarriage as a predictor of obstetric outcome. Obstet Gynecol 2006;107:845–50.
5. Johns J, Jauniaux E. Placental haematomas in early pregnancy. Br J Hosp Med (Lond) 2007;68: 32–5.
6. Deans A, Jauniaux E. Prenatal diagnosis and outcome of subamniotic hematomas. Ultrasound Obstet Gynecol 1998;11:319–23.
7. Jauniaux E, Johns J, Burton GJ. The role of ultrasound imaging in diagnosing and investigating early pregnancy failure. Ultrasound Obstet Gynecol 2005; 25:613–24.
8. Weiss JL, Malone FD, Vidaver J, et al. FASTER Consortium. Threatened abortion: a risk factor for poor pregnancy outcome, a population-based screening study. Am J Obstet Gynecol 2004;190: 745–50.
9. van Oppenraaij RH, Jauniaux E, Christiansen OB, et al. Predicting adverse obstetric outcome after early pregnancy events and complications: a review. Hum Reprod Update 2009;15:409–21.
10. Saraswat L, Bhattacharya S, Maheshwari A, et al. Maternal and perinatal outcome in women with threatened miscarriage in the first trimester: a systematic review. BJOG 2010;117:245–57.
11. Tuuli MG, Norman SM, Odibo AO, et al. Perinatal outcomes in women with subchorionic hematoma: a systematic review and meta-analysis. Obstet Gynecol 2011;117:1205–12.
12. Jauniaux E, Watson AL, Hempstock J, et al. Onset of maternal arterial blood flow and placental oxidative stress; a possible factor in human early pregnancy failure. Am J Pathol 2000;157:2111–22.
13. Jauniaux E, Gulbis B, Burton GJ. The human first trimester gestational sac limits rather than facilitates oxygen transfer to the foetus–a review. Placenta 2003;A:S86–93.
14. Red-Horse K, Zhou Y, Genbacev O, et al. Trophoblast differentiation during embryo implantation

and formation of the maternal-fetal interface. J Clin Invest 2004;114:744–54.

15. Burton GJ. Oxygen, the Janus gas; its effects on human placental development and function. J Anat 2009;215:27–35.

16. Jauniaux E, Greenwold N, Hempstock J, et al. Comparison of ultrasound and Doppler mapping of the intervillous circulation in normal and abnormal early pregnancies. Fertil Steril 2003;79:100–6.

17. Jauniaux E, Hempstock J, Greenwold N, et al. Trophoblastic oxidative stress in relation to temporal and regional differences in maternal placental blood flow in normal and abnormal early pregnancy. Am J Pathol 2003;162:115–25.

18. Burton GJ, Woods AW, Jauniaux E, et al. Rheological and physiological consequences of conversion of the maternal spiral arteries for uteroplacental blood flow during human pregnancy. Placenta 2009;30:473–82.

19. Greenwold N, Jauniaux E, Gulbis B, et al. Relationships between maternal serum, endocrinology, placental karyotype and intervillous circulation in early pregnancy failure. Fertil Steril 2003;79:1373–9.

20. Harville EW, Wilcox AJ, Baird DD, et al. Vaginal bleeding in very early pregnancy. Hum Reprod 2003;18:1944.

21. MbuguaGitau G, Liversedge H, Goffey D, et al. The influence of maternal age on the outcomes of pregnancies complicated by bleeding at less than 12 weeks. Acta Obstet Gynecol Scand 2009;88:116–8.

22. Leite J, Ross P, Rossi AC, et al. Prognosis of very large first-trimester hematomas. J Ultrasound Med 2006;25:1441–5.

23. Maso G, D'Ottavio G, De Seta F, et al. First-trimester intrauterine hematoma and outcome of pregnancy. Obstet Gynecol 2005;105:339–44.

24. Tongsong T, Wanapirak C, Srisomboon J, et al. Transvaginal ultrasound in threatened abortions with empty gestational sacs. Int J Gynaecol Obstet 1994;46(3):297–301.

25. Falco P, Zagonari S, Gabrielli S, et al. Sonography of pregnancies with first-trimester bleeding and a small intrauterine gestational sac without a demonstrable embryo. Ultrasound Obstet Gynecol 2003;21(1):62–5.

26. Nyberg DA, Laing FC, Filly RA. Threatened abortion: sonographic distinction of normal and abnormal gestation sacs. Radiology 1986;158(2):397–400.

27. Elson J, Salim R, Tailor A, et al. Prediction of early pregnancy viability in the absence of an ultrasonically detectable embryo. Ultrasound Obstet Gynecol 2003;21(1):57–61.

28. Mantoni M, Fog Pedersen J. Intrauterine haematoma - an ultrasonic study of threatened abortion. Br J Obstet Gynaecol 1981;88:47–51.

29. Ball RH, Ade CM, Schoenborn JA, et al. The clinical significance of ultrasonographically detected subchorionic haemorrhages. Am J Obstet Gynecol 1996;174:996–1002.

30. Abu-Yousef MM, Bleicher JJ, Williamson RA, et al. Subchorionic hemorrhage: sonographic diagnosis and clinical significance. Am J Roentgenol 1987;149:737.

31. Bennett GL, Bromley B, Lieberman E, et al. Subchorionic haemorrhage in first trimester pregnancies: prediction of pregnancy outcome with sonography. Radiology 1996;200:803–6.

32. Pearlstone M, Baxi L. Subchorionic haematoma: a review. Obstet Gynecol Surv 1993;48:65–8.

33. al-Sebai MA, Diver M, Hipkin LJ. The role of a single free beta-human chorionic gonadotrophin measurement in the diagnosis of early pregnancy failure and the prognosis of fetal viability. Hum Reprod 1996;11(4):881–8.

34. Chung K, Allen R. The use of serial human chorionic gonadotropin levels to establish a viable or a nonviable pregnancy. Semin Reprod Med 2008;26(5):383–90.

35. Duan L, Yan D, Zeng W, et al. Predictive power progesterone combined with beta human chorionic gonadotropin measurements in the outcome of threatened miscarriage. Arch Gynecol Obstet 2011;283(3):431–5.

36. Ruge S, Pedersen JF, Sørensen S, et al. Can pregnancy-associated plasma protein A (PAPP-A) predict the outcome of pregnancy in women with threatened abortion and confirmed fetal viability? Acta Obstet Gynecol Scand 1990;69(7-8):589–95.

37. Johns J, Muttukrishna S, Lygnos M, et al. Maternal serum hormone concentrations for prediction of adverse outcome in threatened miscarriage. Reprod Biomed Online 2007;15(4):413–21.

38. Muttukrishna S, Swer M, Suri S, et al. Soluble Flt-1 and PlGF: new markers of early pregnancy loss? PLoS One 2011;6(3):e18041.

39. Haider S, Knöfler M. Human tumour necrosis factor: physiological and pathological roles in placenta and endometrium. Placenta 2009;30(2):111–23.

40. Hudić I, Fatusić Z. Progesterone-induced blocking factor (PIBF) and Th(1)/Th(2) cytokine in women with threatened spontaneous abortion. J Perinat Med 2009;37(4):338–42.

41. Yamada H, Morikawa M, Furuta I, et al. Circulating cytokines during early pregnancy in women with recurrent spontaneous abortion: decreased TNF-alpha levels in abortion with normal chromosome karyotype. Hokkaido Igaku Zasshi 2004;79(3):237–41.

42. Leal AM, Poon LC, Frisova V, et al. First-trimester maternal serum tumor necrosis factor receptor-1 and pre-eclampsia. Ultrasound Obstet Gynecol 2009;33(2):135–41.

43. Calleja-Agius J, Muttukrishna S, Pizzey AR, et al. Pro- and antiinflammatory cytokines in threatened

miscarriages. Am J Obstet Gynecol 2011. [Epub ahead of print].

44. Bigelow C, Stone J. Bed rest in pregnancy. Mt Sinai J Med 2011;78(2):291–302.

45. Diddle AW, O'Connor KA, Jack R, et al. Evaluation of bed rest in threatened abortion. Obstet Gynecol 1953;2(1):63–7.

46. Ben-Haroush A, Yogev Y, Mashiach R, et al. Pregnancy outcome of threatened abortion with subchorionic hematoma: possible benefit of bed-rest? Isr Med Assoc J 2003;5(6):422–4.

47. Harrison RF. A comparative study of human chorionic gonadotropin, placebo, and bed rest for women with early threatened abortion. Int J Fertil Menopausal Stud 1993;38(3):160–5.

48. Hamilton RA, Grant AM, Henry OA, et al. The management of bleeding in early pregnancy. Ir Med J 1991;84(1):18–9.

49. Aleman A, Althabe F, Belizán J, et al. Bed rest during pregnancy for preventing miscarriage. Cochrane Database Syst Rev 2005;2:CD003576.

50. Wahabi HA, Abed Althagafi NF, Elawad M, et al. Progestogen for treating threatened miscarriage. Cochrane Database Syst Rev 2011;3:CD005943.

51. Gerhard I, Gwinner B, Eggert-Kruse W, et al. Double-blind controlled trial of progesterone substitution in threatened abortion. Biol Res Pregnancy Perinatol 1987;8(1 1ST Half):26–34.

52. Palagiano A, Bulletti C, Pace MC, et al. Effects of vaginal progesterone on pain and uterine contractility in patients with threatened abortion before twelve weeks of pregnancy. Ann N Y Acad Sci 2004;1034:200–10.

53. Devaseelan P, Fogarty PP, Regan L. Human chorionic gonadotrophin for threatened miscarriage. Cochrane Database Syst Rev 2010;5:CD007422.

54. Soltan MH. Buphenine and threatened abortion. Eur J Obstet Gynecol Reprod Biol 1986;22(5-6):319–24.

55. Sotiriadis A, Papatheodorou S, Makrydimas G. Threatened miscarriage: evaluation and management. BMJ 2004;329(7458):152–5.

The Role of First-Trimester Anatomy in Obstetrical Ultrasound

Ori Nevo, MD[a],*, Phyllis Glanc, MD, FRCPC (C)[b]

KEYWORDS

• First trimester • Ultrasound • Obstetrics • Anatomy

Congenital anomalies affecting 2% to 5% of pregnancies are a major cause of infant death and morbidity in North America.[1] Prenatal ultrasound is the most accepted way of detecting fetal anomalies during pregnancy and, once detected, further investigations are instigated, including fetal chromosome analysis; microarray analysis; maternal and fetal investigation for infections; and fetal echocardiogram and magnetic resonance imaging, when indicated, to provide the couple/woman and the health care professional with the full knowledge of the cause, prognosis, and recurrence risk. Common practice is to perform an ultrasound evaluation of fetal anatomy transabdominally at 18 to 22 weeks' gestation.[2,3] The results of the investigations done following this ultrasound may take several weeks. By performing an early anatomy ultrasound, the earlier timeline for diagnosis may give the couple the full spectrum of options for informed decision making.

The performance of early transvaginal anatomy in women who are obese permits bypassing the abdominal pannus, thus, improving image quality as compared with the routine transabdominal approach at 18 to 22 weeks' gestation. The key point of performing an early anatomy ultrasound is to obtain diagnostic information at a time when it is possible to alter the investigation (providing chorionic villus sampling rather than amniocentesis) to provide reassurance of a normally developing pregnancy in the setting of known prior recurrent conditions or under a medical regime that is a risk to the developing fetus. The largest prospective trial to date comparing 12 to 14 weeks' with a 15 to 22 weeks' anatomy examination did not find a detection rate advantage but the distinct ability to provide options for pregnancy management at an earlier date.[4]

The provision of termination at an earlier timeline may reduce physical and psychological morbidity associated with the procedure. The minority of patients with an affected pregnancy will require a high level of expertise and communication skills from their health care team.

A major detractor to the widespread implementation of a transvaginal early anatomy ultrasound is adding an additional examination, thus, placing additional burden on the health care system. For this reason, the examination is recommended to be limited to the indications discussed previously.

The nuchal translucency (NT) scan, which has been introduced as routine screening tool, is performed transabdominally during the first trimester at 11 to 13^{+6} weeks.[5] The primary aim of the NT scan is to assess the maternal risk for fetal chromosomal disorders but not to comprehensively

Disclosures: None.
a Division of Maternal Fetal Medicine, Department of Obstetrics and Gynecology, Sunnybrook Health Sciences Centre, University of Toronto, 2075 Bayview Avenue, Toronto, ON M4N 3M5, Canada
b Abdominal Imaging Division, Department of Medical Imaging, Sunnybrook Health Sciences Centre, University of Toronto, MG104, Sunnybrook Health Sciences Centre, Bayview Campus, 2075 Bayview Avenue, Toronto, ON M4N 3M5 , Canada
* Corresponding author.
E-mail address: ori.nevo@sunnybrook.ca

Ultrasound Clin 7 (2012) 57–73
doi:10.1016/j.cult.2011.11.001
1556-858X/12/$ – see front matter © 2012 Elsevier Inc. All rights reserved.

assess the fetal anatomy. A comprehensive early anatomy ultrasound during the first trimester, which is the focus of this review, is a distinct scan. Although the first-trimester anatomy scan can be performed from about 11 weeks, the suggested optimal time frame to perform an early anatomy ultrasound is at 13 to 15 weeks by a transvaginal approach.

Here, the authors review the present and future role of first-trimester fetal anatomy scan in the obstetric ultrasound.

THE ROUTINE SECOND-TRIMESTER OBSTETRIC SCAN

Ultrasound scanning has become a critical component of antenatal management since the establishment of its diagnostic capabilities in the mid 1970s. Traditionally, and now, the anatomic scan is performed transabdominally at 18 to 22 weeks. However, the optimal timing within the course of a pregnancy to complete the scan continues to be a struggle between the resolution achieved by the ultrasound machine and the gestational age of patients. To accurately assess the anatomic structures of the fetus, the body organs must be large enough to visualize with the resolution of the probe available and must be advanced enough in development to determine whether it is part of the normal development or an abnormality. Schwarzler and colleagues[6] investigated whether any of 3 gestational ages (18, 20, or 22 weeks) was associated with a significant advantage in the detection of fetal anomalies. A total of 1206 patients in an unselected population were evaluated and the end point was defined as the need for a repeat scan because of insufficient anatomic information. This study demonstrated that the later gestational ages, 20 and 22 weeks, had a significantly higher percentage of completed scans (88% and 90%) versus a scan at 18 weeks (76%).[6] The reason for this difference in the completed scan rate was concluded to be caused by the larger size of the body organs that were evaluated.

TRANSVAGINAL EARLY ANATOMY ULTRASOUND

The transvaginal early anatomy ultrasound scan, which is performed at an earlier gestational age (13–16 weeks), is an optimal solution to the conflict between clear visualization and early detection. At 13 to 16 weeks, many of the fetal organs are already fully developed and large enough for viewing and the various fetal body structures can fit into the focal range of the transvaginal transducer.[7]

However, it seems that most studies that examined the detection rate of fetal anomalies during the first trimester were performed during the 11 to 14 weeks' NT scan.[8–10] The detection rate of fetal anomalies was highly variable and ranged between 18%[11] to 54%[12] in the early scan (12–14 weeks) and 48%[11] to 84%[13] in the later scan (18–22 weeks). For example, Taipale and colleagues[11] reported that the detection rate for the early anatomy scan at 13 to 14 weeks in their experience was 18%; in the second scan at 18 to 22 weeks, the detection rate increased to 48%. In comparison, Yagel and colleagues[14] reported in 1995 a detection rate of 83% in early anatomy ultrasound performed at 13 to 16 weeks. At least half of the nondetected anomalies in this study are known to present later in pregnancy (mainly brain abnormalities, such as hydrocephaly or agenesis of corpus callosum).

The reason for the differences in the detection rate between the various studies is likely because of the variation in terms of gestational age at the first-trimester evaluation, technique and machine used (transabdominal vs transvaginal), and sonographer training and experience.

ROLE OF SONOGRAPHER EXPERIENCE IN EARLY ANATOMY ULTRASOUND

The examiner's expertise in performing the early anatomy examination is of the utmost importance. Early anatomy ultrasound is not performed routinely; thus, most sonographers are not trained in the examination. Additionally, several fetal organs (such as the cerebellum and vermis)[15] seem undeveloped during the first trimester and gain their final shape only later in pregnancy, thus, necessitating further knowledge and experience in early fetal anatomy. Taipale and colleagues[16] have shown that there is a learning curve in ultrasound detection of fetal anomalies in early pregnancies at 13 to 14 weeks. Although the detection rate was only 22% during the beginning of their study, it increased to 79% during the fourth year of the study. Bronshtein and Zimmer[17] have emphasized the importance of experience and training in early ultrasound, suggesting that a high detection rate is more likely after proper training.

The Society of Obstetricians and Gynecologist in Canada has also recognized the importance of experience as reflected in the guideline, "*Women at increased risk of fetal structural and genetic abnormalities should be offered such screening, performed by an experienced sonologist.*"[18] The authors support the previous literature and guidelines and suggest that both technologists and physicians have training and experience in first-trimester anatomy scans before performing it independently for clinical purposes.

PREFERRED TECHNIQUE FOR FIRST-TRIMESTER ANATOMY ULTRASOUND

The routine second-trimester anatomy scan is performed transabdominally because the fetal size is large enough and detailed anatomy is seen with acceptable resolution. During the first trimester, the fetal size is small, with maximal crown rump length (CRL) of 80 mm at 14 weeks and the uterus is still located in the lower pelvis. Therefore, the transabdominal approach is suboptimal in most cases, and the transvaginal approach with a high-frequency and high-resolution probe provides more detailed anatomic information as suggested by several studies.[17,19]

Rosati and colleagues[19] reported that transabdominal anatomic evaluation at 15 weeks was completed in 50% of cases, whereas transvaginally, a complete scan was achieved in 85% of cases. In contrast, Braithwaite and colleagues[20] reported that a complete anatomic survey was achieved in 95% of fetuses at 12 to 13 weeks, and a transvaginal approach was used in only 20% of cases. However, the protocol used did not include a detailed anatomy of the face, ears, and digits. Souka and colleagues[21] reported the use of both transabdominal and transvaginal approaches for the detection of structural anomalies at 11 to 14 weeks. The sensitivity of the early scan in the detection of major structural anomalies was 50% and increased to 92% at the second scan at 22 to 24 weeks. The same group also reported that the use of a transvaginal approach increased the completeness of the examination from 72% to 86% and was helpful in examining the face, kidneys, and bladder.[22] Braithwaite[23] addressed concerns regarding the acceptability and discomfort of transvaginal ultrasound. Marked discomfort was reported by 0.7% of patients, and 95% reported that they would have no concerns having an additional transvaginal ultrasound, suggesting that vaginal ultrasound is acceptable and is not associated with unusual discomfort.

TIMING OF EARLY ANATOMY ULTRASOUND

The timing of performing an early anatomy scan is important and may affect the completeness of the examination and the detection rate. Rosati and colleagues[19] showed that the visualization rate of complete fetal anatomy increased with gestational age and concluded that a detailed evaluation of fetal anatomy is possible in most cases at 13 weeks. Souka and colleagues[22] have reported that visualization of fetal anatomy improved with increasing gestational age when examining the fetal anatomy during NT. Because a complete scan at 13 weeks could be achieved in 98% of patients, they concluded that the optimal gestational age to examine fetal anatomy in the first trimester is 13 weeks. Monteagudo and Timor-Tritsch[24] have suggested that fetal anatomy can be adequately evaluated at 12 weeks and ideally between 13 to 14 weeks. Because a subset of fetal anomalies may not be present during the first trimester, all studies suggest a follow-up anatomic scan at 20 to 23 weeks.[14,24]

FIRST-TRIMESTER ANATOMY: TO WHOM?

Despite the high detection rate of a transvaginal early anatomy scan, the current practice in Canada and in most countries is to perform a transabdominal ultrasound scan to evaluate fetal anatomy at 18 to 22 weeks' of gestation for both low-risk and at-risk patients. This practice leads to delay in diagnosis and management of patients with fetal anomalies as reflected by the data from The Fetal Alert Network, which reported that mean gestational age of initial diagnosis of fetal anomalies in Ontario, Canada is at 21 weeks and the mean time of referral to a high-risk service is 24.6 weeks.[25]

Hypothetically, a first-trimester anatomy scan would be of benefit for the general obstetric population. However, because of limited resources and especially when first-trimester anatomy is performed as a separate scan in addition to the routine NT scan, it is not feasible in many countries. Therefore, it is suggested to perform a first-trimester anatomy scan to patients who are at risk and will benefit the most. The following subpopulations are considered at risk: (1) increased fetal NT[26,27]; (2) known parental-inherited conditions associated with fetal abnormalities; (3) previous pregnancy with fetal abnormalities that are associated with an increased risk for fetal anomalies in the present pregnancy; (4) maternal exposures or diseases, such as infection; and (5) patients who are prone to have an incomplete anatomy scan at 18 to 22 weeks because of significant obesity or abdominal wall scars that impede sound transmission.[28] Early detection of fetal anomalies in this subgroup of women would not only provide women with more options regarding the management of their pregnancy but also might reduce stress levels during the pregnancy when the fetal anatomy is normal as is expected in most cases.

ROLE OF FIRST-TRIMESTER ANATOMY IN WOMEN WHO ARE OBESE

Obesity has become common in our society and has important implications for pregnancy and obstetric ultrasound. It is estimated that obesity, as defined by body mass index (BMI) greater than or equal to 30, is found in up to 30% of North American women of child-bearing age.[29]

Interestingly, it has been shown that the risk for congenital anomalies is increased in women who are obese, but the cause is unknown.[30] Watkins and colleagues[31] reported that women who are obese have a 3.5-fold increase in the risk for neural tube defect, a 3.3-fold increased risk for omphalocele, and a 2-fold increase in the risk for cardiac anomaly and for multiple anomalies. This observation is supported by other studies that have demonstrated that maternal obesity is associated with an increased risk for fetal structural anomalies, with specific risk for anomalies of the spine, heart, and abdominal wall.[30,32,33]

Although ultrasound technology has evolved, sonographic visualization of fetal anatomic structures continues to be negatively affected by maternal obesity, and image quality is diminished in women with a thick abdominal wall.[34,35] Hendler and colleagues[28] have shown that, not surprisingly, the quality of the anatomic scan is decreased in patients who are obese and, in fact, there is a correlation between the level of obesity and the ability to complete the scan. Cardiac anatomy, which is an important part of a routine anatomy scan but more so in women who are obese, was not properly seen at 18 weeks in 23% of patients who were obese with a BMI greater than 30, thus, curtailing the ability to detect cardiac anomalies at this point.[36] Maxwell and colleagues[37] reported that the anatomy scan was incomplete in 26.0% of women who were obese compared with only 2.5% in nonobese patients. Studies have demonstrated that not only does maternal obesity affect image quality but, consequently, the ability to detect structural anomalies is significantly reduced: a 42% detection rate versus 86% detection rate in a nonobese population.[38]

The projected benefit of a transvaginal early ultrasound scan in women who are obese is clear. This approach would avoid the obstacle of a thickened abdominal wall and could potentially increase the quality of images obtained and the detection rate of anomalies in this subpopulation. The authors have piloted this approach in their high-risk referral clinic with a group of 29 women with a BMI greater than or equal to 30 Kg/m^2 that were screened for fetal anatomic abnormalities using early transvaginal ultrasound. The authors completed a full early anatomy ultrasound in 82% of the patients at 12 to 15 weeks. The quality of the images was superior to the quality achieved by the routine transabdominal scan at 18 to 22 weeks, and fetal abnormalities were detected in 5 patients.[39] These findings suggest that early anatomy may have an important role in the management of pregnancies in women who are obese.

ROLE OF 3-DIMENSIONAL ULTRASOUND IN FIRST-TRIMESTER ANATOMY

The availability of 3-dimensional (3D) ultrasound is intriguing when attempting to examine fetal anatomy during the first trimester. The fetus is relatively small during the first trimester and, thus, it is possible to acquire the whole fetus in a limited number of 3D acquisitions. Once the volumes are acquired, they can be examined off line by physicians who are experienced in manipulation of 3D volumes and interpretation of first-trimester anatomy. Michailidis and colleagues[40] reported one of the first studies that aimed to explore the feasibility of performing a complete anatomic scan of the fetus at 12 to 13 weeks using transvaginally acquired 3D volumes. Excluding cardiac anatomy, a complete anatomic scan was achieved in 80% of cases using 3D alone. Fauchon and colleagues[41] attempted to examine whether a basic fetal anatomy scan can be performed during an NT scan at 11 to 13 + 6 weeks using transabdominal 3D volumes. A total of 40% to 90% of listed organs were seen. Not surprisingly, there was a positive correlation of success rate and CRL and lower success in correlation to maternal weight. Of note, the study focused on the Fetal Medicine Foundation guidelines, and it was not aimed to perform a full anatomy scan.

There are 2 more recent studies that examined the visualization rate of fetal anatomy using 3D ultrasound. Bhaduri and colleagues[42] examined fetal anatomy at 12 to 13 weeks using five 3D volumes. The head and abdomen were seen in almost all fetuses, but skin above the lower spine and the heart was seen in 26% to 18% of fetuses. A complete anatomic survey was achieved in up to 33% at 13 weeks. Antsaklis and colleagues[43] have recently reported that using transabdominal 3D acquisitions, the fetal head, abdomen, stomach, and limbs were identified in 87% to 93% of cases, whereas the bladder, heart, and face were seen in 57% to 82% of cases. Both studies concluded that 3D ultrasound for visualization of fetal anatomy during the NT scan is insufficient to evaluate several major organs and, therefore, is not reliable as a single method to assess fetal anatomy during the first trimester. Additionally, all previous studies have not reported the detection rate of fetal anomalies by first-trimester 3D scan, which is the main purpose of performing an anatomic scan during pregnancy.

FETAL ANOMALIES

The whole spectrum of detectable fetal anomalies during the first trimester is too wide to be included in this short review. Therefore, the authors have elected to focus on organ systems that are associated with the more common anomalies and have major impact on the expected outcome of the fetus, such as the cardiovascular system, central nervous system, and musculoskeletal disorders. The authors present cases from their own experience that likely represent the more common fetal anomalies presenting to a high-risk referral service.

CENTRAL NERVOUS SYSTEM
Embryology

The brain develops from the neural fold that forms 3 primary vesicles: prosencephalon, mesencephalon, and rhombencephalon. During the fifth week of gestation, the primary vesicles divide into secondary vesicles forming the telencephalon and the diencephalon. The hindbrain divides into the metencephalon and myelencephalon. During the fourth week, the brain forms the midbrain flexure and cervical flexure, whereas the pontine flexure appears later.

The myelencephalon vesicle forms the adult medulla and lower part of the fourth ventricle. The metencephalon forms the pons and cerebellum and upper part of the fourth ventricle. The cerebellum develops during the end of the fifth week from posterior swellings that enlarge and fuse in the median plane. The forebrain gives rise to the optic vesicles, which later form the retinas and optic nerves. The telencephalic vesicles form the cerebral hemispheres and the lateral ventricles, whereas the third ventricle is formed mainly by the diencephalon. Expansion of the cerebral hemispheres makes them cover the diencephalon midbrain and hindbrain.

The corpus callosum is the most important commissure and begins its development at 10 weeks when fibers cross the lamina terminalis and connects the two hemispheres.

The surface of the cerebral hemispheres is smooth during the first trimester, and sulci and gyri develop later during the second and third trimesters.

Sonography of Normal Brain

The early fetal brain is examined in multiple transverse sections as depicted in **Fig. 1**. The brain seems relatively simplified compared with the fetal brain during the late second trimester because the brain has not completed its structural development. The falx cerebri symmetrically divides the space in two. The choroid plexus seems prominent and fills the mid and posterior part of the lateral ventricles. The third ventricle can be seen between the thalami, and the midline aqueduct may be seen in its course toward the fourth ventricle. In the posterior fossa, the cerebellum and upper vermis are seen. The lower vermis is undeveloped, and a small connection between the fourth ventricle and the small cisterna magna is normally seen at this stage.

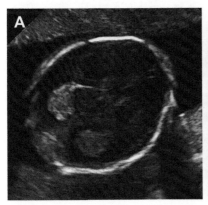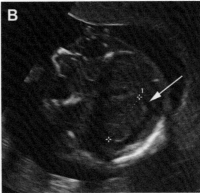

Fig. 1. Normal fetal brain at 14 weeks. (*A*) Transverse view at the level of the lateral ventricles. The choroid occupies the ventricular space and the cortex is relatively thin. Midline falx is present. (*B*) Low transverse view showing the posterior fossa and cerebellum (*arrow*), orbits, and nasal bones.

Congenital Anomalies

Brain development is a complex process; therefore, brain anomalies are common as isolated disorders or as part of multiple anomalies and are estimated as 3 per 1000 birth.

ANENCEPHALY

This condition is common and can be detected during the first trimester (**Fig. 2**). The main characteristics of anencephaly are absent of normal cranium and telencephalon. The diagnosis can be made at 11 to 12 weeks when absent skull calcification is seen and the unsupported brain floats in the amniotic fluid.[44] The disintegration of the brain forms the pathognomonic milky appearance of the amniotic fluid. The cause of the condition is multifactorial and is considered to be a form of abnormal closure of the anterior neuropore and can be associated with other anomalies, such as spina bifida, facial clefts, clubfoot, or omphalocele.

OCCIPITAL BONE PROTUBERANCE

The authors have recently reported the occurrence of transient occipital bone protuberance during the first trimester, which is characterized by a small, bony protuberance (2–3 mm) with no cerebral tissue involvement and is located in the midline or paramedian occipital bone (**Fig. 3**). The cause of this finding is not completely known, but the authors have speculated that overlapping cranial bones; wormian bone; or local lesion, such as epidermoid or hemangioma, may be the cause. The protuberance was not seen during a repeat scan at 19 to 24 weeks, and the outcome was normal in all cases.[45]

HYDROCEPHALY

Hydrocephaly is defined as progressive increase in ventricular volume caused by obstruction between cerebral spaces. Other forms of dilated ventricles from other causes are referred to as ventriculomegaly. Early hydrocephaly has been reported from 13 weeks onward as shown in **Fig. 4**. The early sign of hydrocephaly is the island sign, which indicates separation of the choroid plexus from the ventricular wall of the lateral ventricles. However, only the minority of cases with island sign will continue and progress to overt hydrocephaly or alternatively be associated with mild transient ventriculomegaly.[44]

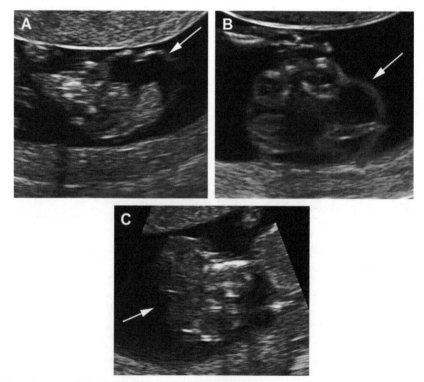

Fig. 2. Acrania and exencephaly. (*A*) Exencephaly at 11 weeks: disorganized brain tissue surrounded by covering membrane (*arrow*). (*B*) Acrania at 12 weeks: no calcified skull bones were detected (*arrow*). (*C*) Exencephaly at 10 weeks (*arrow*).

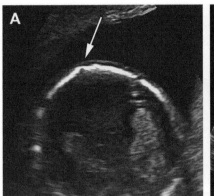
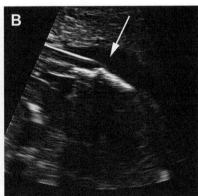

Fig. 3. Transient occipital protuberance. Transverse (*A*) and sagittal (*B*) views of a fetal head showing a small protuberance of the occipital bone (*arrow*). The finding disappeared by 19 weeks with normal outcome at birth.

MIDLINE ANOMALIES
Holoprosencephaly

It is thought that failure in the normal division of the prosencephalon is the underlying cause of midline anomalies, such as holoprosencephaly (HPE). Traditionally, 3 forms of holoprosencephaly are described and correspond to the severity of the disorder: lobar, semilobar, and alobar HPE. Another form of HPE is the midline interhemispheric HPE or syntelencephaly, which is less common than the other forms.

In semilobar and lobar HPE, there is a midline single ventricle with a variable degree of microcephaly or macrocephaly caused by hydrocephaly. HPE is commonly associated with facial anomalies, such as hypotelorism, cyclopia, facial clefts, and nasal anomalies, and is known to be part of chromosomal disorders, such as triploidy and trisomy 13 and 18.[44]

The disorder can be diagnosed very early during the first trimester, and the main features are a single midline ventricle with absent separation of the 2 cerebral hemispheres (**Fig. 5**) and various facial anomalies.

ANOMALIES OF THE CORPUS CALLOSUM

The corpus callosum is the main commissure connecting the 2 hemispheres. The development of the corpus callosum begins at 10 to 12 weeks; therefore, anomalies of the corpus callosum are not readily diagnosed during the first trimester. However, there are several sonographic findings during the first trimester that can be the first sign of agenesis of corpus callosum (ACC), such as dilation of the third ventricle (**Fig. 6**) with splayed thalami.

POSTERIOR FOSSA
Dandy Walker Malformation

Dandy Walker (DW) malformation is commonly defined as the complete or partial agenesis of the cerebellar vermis, cystic dilatation of the fourth

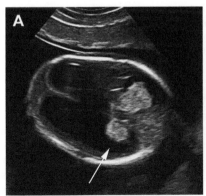
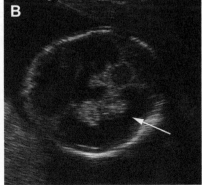

Fig. 4. Hydrocephaly. Two cases of hydrocephaly at 13 to 14 weeks. (*A*) Note the dilated lateral ventricles with disruption of the interhemispheric septum and dilated third ventricle (*B*). The choroid plexus (*arrow*) is abnormally floating in the ventricle.

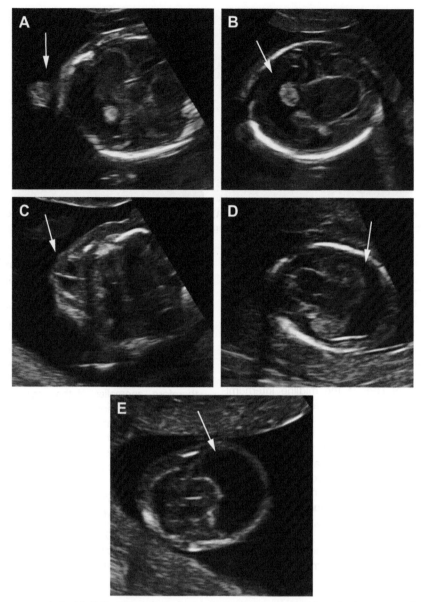

Fig. 5. Holoprosencephaly. (*A–C*) Semilobar holoprosencephaly associated with cyclopia at 14 weeks. Proboscis is seen in (*A*) and the midline single orbit in (*C*). (*D*) Semilobar holoprosencephaly at 13 weeks. (*E*) Alobar holoprosencephaly at 12 weeks: the characteristic absence of the midline structures (falx, interhemispheric fissure) and a primitive single ventricle (*arrow*) with fusion of the thalami.

ventricle, and enlargement of the posterior fossa with upward displacement of the tentorium. Hydrocephaly is a common complication of the disorder and is present in many but not all of the cases. The features of DW malformation can be observed during the late first trimester with enlargement of the cisterna magna and a large defect in the posterior cerebellum (**Fig. 7**).

Although most brain anomalies can be detected during the first trimester, there are a subset of disorders, such as late onset hydrocephaly, ACC, microcephaly, craniosynostosis, and others, that may appear only after 18 to 20 weeks. Therefore, a repeat brain anatomy scan at 19 to 23 weeks is recommended for patients who have a first-trimester anatomy.

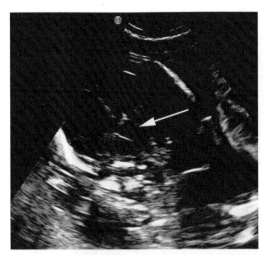

Fig. 6. Dilated third ventricle with splayed thalami (*arrow*) at 14+ weeks. The fetus later developed mild ventriculomegaly and hypoplastic corpus callosum at 19 weeks.

CARDIOVASCULAR SYSTEM
Embryology

During the late third week of fetal development, the angioblastic cords canalize and fuse to form the tubular heart. Heartbeats begin at 22 to 23 days, and blood flow appears during the fourth week. The primordial myocardium develops around the endothelial tube, which will form the endocardium. The bulbus cordis and ventricle grow faster than other parts of the heart and bend to form the bulboventricular loop. The endocardial cushions develop during the end of the fourth week to form the walls of the atrioventricular (AV) canal. Later, the cushions fuse and separate the canal to right and left and will form the AV valves and membranous septa. The atria are separated by the septum primum that originate in the roof of the atrium. The septum secundum develop from the cranial wall of the atria to the right of the septum primum. This septum grows during the fifth and sixth week and overlaps the foramen secundum. The ventricles are separated by a muscular patch that arises from the floor of the ventricle and is extended during the growth of the ventricles. The interventricular septum closes by the end of the seventh week by the formation of the membranous part of the septum. The great arteries develop from the bulbus cordis and truncus arteriosus during the fifth and sixth weeks of development. Bulbar and truncal ridges develop and form the spiral aorticopulmonary septum, which divides the aorta and pulmonary trunk. This process is completed by 7 weeks' of development and, thus, by 8 weeks' of development (equivalent to 10 weeks' of gestation) the cardiac structural development is complete and can be assessed during the first trimester (**Fig. 8**).[46]

CARDIAC ANOMALIES

Congenital heart disease is one of the common congenital anomalies and occurs in 6 to 8 per 1000 births.[47] The condition may be associated with other anomalies, chromosomal disorders, and substantial postnatal morbidity. Therefore, prenatal diagnosis is important for proper counseling and planning the management during pregnancy and delivery.

HYPOPLASTIC LEFT HEART SYNDROME

Hypoplastic left heart syndrome (HLHS) is defined when the left ventricle is hypoplastic and is associated with severe stenosis or atresia of the mitral valve and the aortic outflow tract (**Fig. 9**). HLHS includes a spectrum of presentations: from severe aortic stenosis with mildly smaller left ventricle (LV) to more severe forms with atretic mitral valve and aorta and extremely small LV. In cases whereby there is no forward flow in the ascending aorta, a retrograde blood flow from the ductus arteriosus is evident in the aortic arch (see **Fig. 9**). Most cases of HLHS can be diagnosed during the first trimester, although in some cases, the first presentation is of aortic coarctation and mild asymmetry between the ventricles that progresses during the second trimester to the classic HLHS.[48]

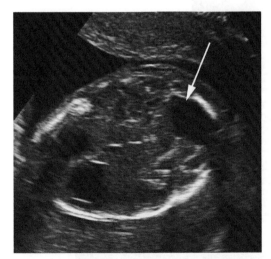

Fig. 7. DW malformation at 13 weeks. Large posterior fossa cyst with splaying of the hypoplastic cerebellar hemispheres (*arrow*). The fetus had increased NT and was found to have Turner syndrome.

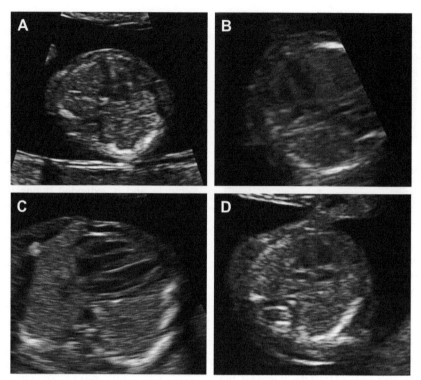

Fig. 8. Normal 4-chamber view during the first trimester. (*A*, *B*) Normal heart at 12 weeks. (*C*, *D*) A 14 weeks' heart. Perpendicular view of the septum at 14 weeks (*C*) with detailed view of the atrioventricular valves apparatus.

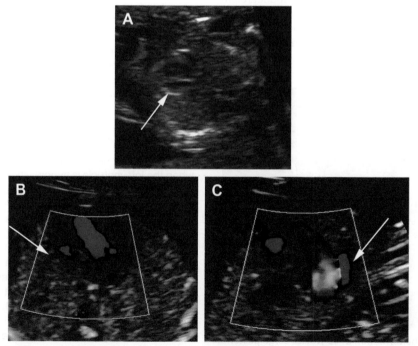

Fig. 9. Hypoplastic left heart syndrome. (*A*) HLHS at 13 weeks with a markedly small left ventricle compared with the right ventricle. (*B*, *C*) HLHS at 14+ weeks showing a very small left ventricle and retrograde flow in the aortic arch (*C*).

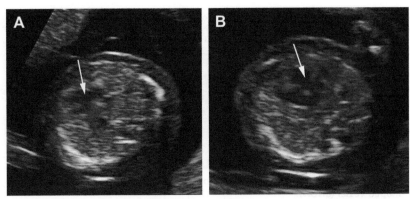

Fig. 10. Atrioventricular septal defect. (A) Large defect at the level of the AV valves (arrow) at 12 weeks. (B) Linear insertion of AV valves with large defect in the interventricular septum (arrow) at 12 weeks. Both fetuses had diffuse skin edema and were found to have trisomy 21.

ATRIOVENTRICULAR SEPTAL DEFECT

Atrioventricular septal defect (AVSD) is defined as the incomplete development of the inferior aspect of septum primum, the endocardial cushion, and the AV valves. The disorder includes a spectrum of anomalies with various degrees of severity and is associated with chromosomal disorders and primarily Down syndrome in more than half of the cases.[49]

The main sonographic signs of AVSD are linear insertion of the AV valves, defect at the level of AV valves with shared inflow, and unstable crux (Fig. 10).[50]

TETRALOGY OF FALLOT

The characteristic findings of tetralogy of Fallot (TOF) can be seen during the first trimester; overriding aorta, ventricular septal defect, pulmonary

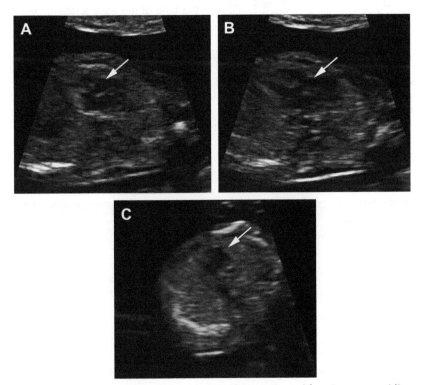

Fig. 11. TOF. (A, B) The aorta is overlapping the interventricular septum and forming an overriding aorta (arrow). (C) Three-vessel view showing a markedly large aorta compared with the smaller pulmonary artery (arrow).

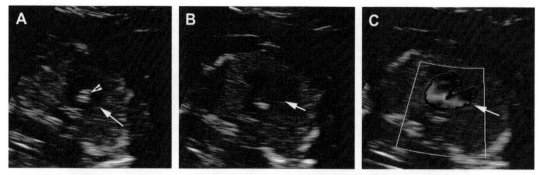

Fig. 12. Right aortic arch at 14 weeks. The trachea (*arrow head*) is encircled by the elongated right aortic arch that forms a U-shaped vessel (*arrow*).

stenosis, although hypertrophy of the right ventricle is the hallmarks of TOF, although the latest is usually not apparent prenatally (**Fig. 11**).

RIGHT AORTIC ARCH

Abnormal development of the aortic arch may result in a right or double aortic arch that forms vascular rings around the trachea and esophagus. Prenatal diagnosis of vascular band during the first trimester was reported before.[51] The main hallmarks are visualization of an artery surrounding the trachea, which is usually associated with a right aortic arch. A right aortic arch is longer than a normal arch and makes its turn on the right side (**Fig. 12**).

ABSENT DUCTUS VENOSUS

Absence of the ductus venosus is a rare disorder and may be associated with other fetal anomalies or chromosomal disorders. The abnormal venous return leads to increase flow through the liver or to the right atrium and may induce fetal hydrops.[52] Prenatal diagnosis during the first trimester has

been reported and is characterized in most cases by abnormal course of the intrahepatic umbilical vein, which is connected to the inferior vena cava (IVC), right atrium, or other large veins (**Figs. 13–15**).

Musculoskeletal Fetal Dysplasias

Skeletal dysplasias represent a heterogeneous group of bone disorders. The overall incidence is approximately 2.4/100,000 births, excluding limb amputations, thus, accounting for approximately 5% of congenital neonatal abnormalities.[53] The prevalence of musculoskeletal fetal dysplasias at the time of the early anatomic evaluation has not yet been determined.

Both the 11- to 14-week examination and the early transvaginal anatomic evaluation (13–15 weeks) are good times to evaluate the fetal skeleton because bone ossification is complete by 11 weeks' gestational age (**Figs. 16** and **17**).[54,55] First-trimester and early second-trimester fetal limb length charts are available for reference.[56–58] As in a diagnosis performed at later stages of pregnancy, detailed anatomic

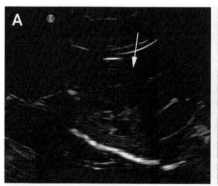
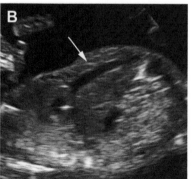

Fig. 13. Case of absent ductus venosus at 14 weeks. (*A*) The umbilical vein is connecting directly to the right atrium (*arrow*). (*B*) The abnormal course of the umbilical vein in the anterior abdomen (*arrow*).

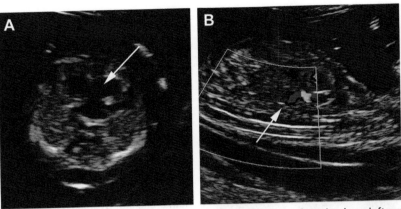

Fig. 14. Left isomerism. A case of a 13-week fetus with increased NT that was found to have left cardiac isomerism and bradycardia. (*A*) Symmetric ventricles with large AVSD (*arrow*). (*B*) Interrupted inferior vena cava (*arrow*).

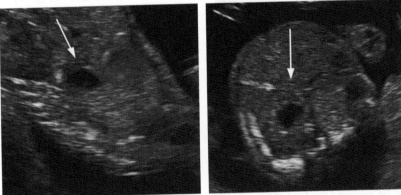

Fig. 15. Congenital diaphragmatic hernia at 14 weeks. The stomach and bowel (*arrow*) are in the left chest with absence of left-side diaphragm. The more echogenic right lung is seen in the right chest. We have diagnosed other anomalies that were associated with increased NT such as left cardiac isomerism (**Fig. 14**) and diaphragmatic hernia (**Fig. 15**).

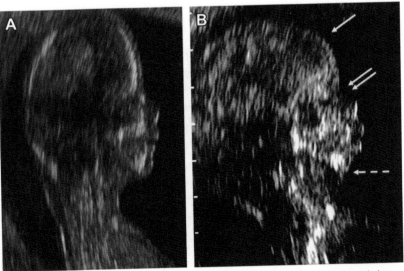

Fig. 16. A 14 weeks' gestational age fetus with profile image. (*A*) Normal. (*B*) Osteogenesis imperfecta type 2A. Note absent cranial vault ossification (*arrow*), absent nasal bone ossification (*double arrow*), and retrognathia (*dashed arrow*).

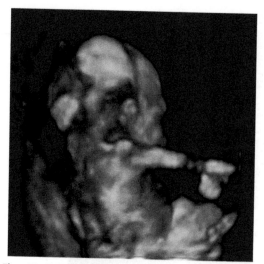

Fig. 17. A 3D-rendered image at 13 weeks' gestational age of fetus with radial ray aplasia. The skeletal system is ideally suited to 3D-rendered images in view of the high contrast and early ossification.

between them, similar to later in gestation (Fig. 18).[59] Increased NT is a common feature of serious lethal skeletal dysplasias, suggesting that the presence of an enlarged NT or hydrops fetalis is an indication for the evaluation of the musculoskeletal system.[60–62]

There are several publications indicating the ability of early diagnosis of fetal musculoskeletal disorders but the most compelling is a recent publication that retrospectively analyzed more than 45,000 singleton pregnancies at the 11 to 13+ weeks scan and identified most cases of a missing hand or foot (77.8%), about half of the lethal skeletal dysplasias and isolated long bone hypoplasia and polydactyl cases, 25.0% bilateral talipes, and 3.8% unilateral talipes. A significant increase in the incidence of NT more than the 95th percentile was noted in lethal skeletal dysplasias and bilateral talipes, suggesting that there may be a role for skeletal evaluation in the setting of increased NT.[63] In lethal skeletal dysplasias, early termination may actually impede the ability to diagnose the condition, thus, limiting counseling for future pregnancies. The primary role of early anatomic diagnosis is to predict lethality. Secondary goals are to determine the diagnosis or narrow the differential diagnosis. The lethal group of skeletal dysplasias typically has an earlier onset with more severe phenotypic features than the nonlethal group, thus, lethal skeletal dysplasias are potentially more amenable to early diagnosis.[64,65] After birth, postnatal radiographs, autopsy (in lethal cases), and molecular testing are critical to obtaining a specific diagnosis.[66–69]

evaluation, accurate postnatal evaluation, and genetic consultation are required to confirm diagnosis and counseling. Accurate specific diagnosis tends to be made in cases presenting with a known family history. For most cases, postnatal imaging, pathology, karyotype, and molecular diagnosis may be required for final diagnosis. Of the common lethal skeletal dysplasias, the shared features are small chest and micromelia, whereas the presence of abnormal mineralization, fractures, and macrocranium may help to distinguish

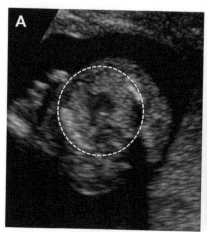
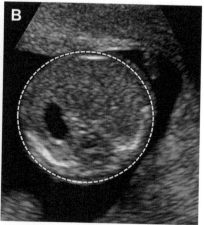

Fig. 18. Small thorax diagnosed at 13 weeks in case of dyssegmental dysplasia. The chest circumference (white circle) is significantly smaller than the abdominal circumference (white circle). (A) Cross-section of the thorax. (B) Cross-section of the abdomen.

SUMMARY

The human fetus reaches major developmental milestones during the first trimester of pregnancy, and most of the known birth defects appear during this time. Late first-trimester ultrasound is highly effective in detecting congenital malformations when performed transvaginally by experienced operators. Although the first-trimester anatomy scan has not been introduced as a routine examination in most countries, it is recommended to patients at risk for having fetal anomalies and likely helpful in women who are obese in an attempt to improve the quality of the images and improve the timely detection of congenital anomalies. Further development of 3D ultrasound technologies may prove to be efficacious in future first-trimester anatomy scans and may be incorporated with the NT scan, although the 2-dimensional ultrasound is currently the preferred technique.

REFERENCES

1. Yoon PW, Olney RS, Khoury MJ, et al. Contribution of birth defects and genetic diseases to pediatric hospitalizations. A population-based study. Arch Pediatr Adolesc Med 1997;151:1096–103.
2. Cargill Y, Morin L, Bly S, et al. Content of a complete routine second trimester obstetrical ultrasound examination and report. J Obstet Gynaecol Can 2009;31:272–80.
3. ACOG Practice Bulletin No. 101: ultrasonography in pregnancy. Obstet Gynecol 2009;113:451–61.
4. Saltvedt S, Almstrom H, Kublickas M, et al. Detection of malformations in chromosomally normal fetuses by routine ultrasound at 12 or 18 weeks of gestation-a randomised controlled trial in 39,572 pregnancies. BJOG 2006;113:664–74.
5. Nicolaides KH. Screening for fetal aneuploidies at 11 to 13 weeks. Prenat Diagn 2011;31:7–15.
6. Schwarzler P, Senat MV, Holden D, et al. Feasibility of the second-trimester fetal ultrasound examination in an unselected population at 18, 20 or 22 weeks of pregnancy: a randomized trial. Ultrasound Obstet Gynecol 1999;14:92–7.
7. Timor-Tritsch IE. As technology evolves, so should its application: shortcomings of the "18-week anatomy scan". J Ultrasound Med 2006;25:423–8.
8. Carvalho MH, Brizot ML, Lopes LM, et al. Detection of fetal structural abnormalities at the 11-14 week ultrasound scan. Prenat Diagn 2002;22:1–4.
9. Fong KW, Toi A, Hornberger LK, et al. Detection of fetal structural abnormalities with US during early pregnancy. Radiographics 2004;24:157–74.
10. Rottem S, Bronshtein M. Transvaginal sonographic diagnosis of congenital anomalies between 9 weeks and 16 weeks, menstrual age. J Clin Ultrasound 1990;18:307–14.
11. Taipale P, Ammala M, Salonen R, et al. Two-stage ultrasonography in screening for fetal anomalies at 13-14 and 18-22 weeks of gestation. Acta Obstet Gynecol Scand 2004;83:1141–6.
12. Chen M, Lam YH, Lee CP, et al. Ultrasound screening of fetal structural abnormalities at 12 to 14 weeks in Hong Kong. Prenat Diagn 2004;24:92–7.
13. Guariglia L, Rosati P. Transvaginal sonographic detection of embryonic-fetal abnormalities in early pregnancy. Obstet Gynecol 2000;96:328–32.
14. Yagel S, Achiron R, Ron M, et al. Transvaginal ultrasonography at early pregnancy cannot be used alone for targeted organ ultrasonographic examination in a high-risk population. Am J Obstet Gynecol 1995;172:971–5.
15. Bromley B, Nadel AS, Pauker S, et al. Closure of the cerebellar vermis: evaluation with second trimester US. Radiology 1994;193:761–3.
16. Taipale P, Ammala M, Salonen R, et al. Learning curve in ultrasonographic screening for selected fetal structural anomalies in early pregnancy. Obstet Gynecol 2003;101:273–8.
17. Bronshtein M, Zimmer EZ. Prenatal ultrasound examinations: for whom, by whom, what, when and how many? Ultrasound Obstet Gynecol 1997;10:1–4.
18. Demianczuk NN, Van Den Hof MC, Farquharson D, et al. The use of first trimester ultrasound. J Obstet Gynaecol Can 2003;25(10):864–75.
19. Rosati P, Guariglia L, Bertuzzi A. Transvaginal assessment of fetal anatomy at 11 to 16 weeks of gestation in relation to fetal position. Fetal Diagn Ther 2000;15:63–70.
20. Braithwaite JM, Armstrong MA, Economides DL. Assessment of fetal anatomy at 12 to 13 weeks of gestation by transabdominal and transvaginal sonography. Br J Obstet Gynaecol 1996;103:82–5.
21. Souka AP, Pilalis A, Kavalakis I, et al. Screening for major structural abnormalities at the 11- to 14-week ultrasound scan. Am J Obstet Gynecol 2006;194:393–6.
22. Souka AP, Pilalis A, Kavalakis Y, et al. Assessment of fetal anatomy at the 11-14-week ultrasound examination. Ultrasound Obstet Gynecol 2004;24:730–4.
23. Braithwaite JM, Economides DL. Acceptability by patients of transvaginal sonography in the elective assessment of the first-trimester fetus. Ultrasound Obstet Gynecol 1997;9:91–3.
24. Monteagudo A, Timor-Tritsch IE. First trimester anatomy scan: pushing the limits. What can we see now? Curr Opin Obstet Gynecol 2003;15:131–41.
25. Windrim R. Fetal Alert Network: a need for a population based antenatal network. Am J Obstet Gynecol 2006;195:S219.

26. Adekunle O, Gopee A, el Sayed M, et al. Increased first trimester nuchal translucency: pregnancy and infant outcomes after routine screening for Down's syndrome in an unselected antenatal population. Br J Radiol 1999;72:457–60.

27. Devine PC, Simpson LL. Nuchal translucency and its relationship to congenital heart disease. Semin Perinatol 2000;24:343–51.

28. Hendler I, Blackwell SC, Bujold E, et al. Suboptimal second-trimester ultrasonographic visualization of the fetal heart in obese women: should we repeat the examination? J Ultrasound Med 2005;24:1205–9.

29. Ogden CL, Carroll MD. Prevalence of overweight, obesity, and extreme obesity among adults: United States, trends 1960–1962 through 2007–2008. Centers for Disease Control and Prevention. National Center for Health Statistics. June 2010.

30. Waller DK, Mills JL, Simpson JL, et al. Are obese women at higher risk for producing malformed offspring? Am J Obstet Gynecol 1994;170:541–8.

31. Watkins ML, Rasmussen SA, Honein MA, et al. Maternal obesity and risk for birth defects. Pediatrics 2003;111:1152–8.

32. Mikhail LN, Walker CK, Mittendorf R. Association between maternal obesity and fetal cardiac malformations in African Americans. J Natl Med Assoc 2002;94:695–700.

33. Watkins ML, Botto LD. Maternal prepregnancy weight and congenital heart defects in offspring. Epidemiology 2001;12:439–46.

34. Rosenberg JC, Guzman ER, Vintzileos AM, et al. Transumbilical placement of the vaginal probe in obese pregnant women. Obstet Gynecol 1995;85: 132–4.

35. Wolfe HM, Sokol RJ, Martier SM, et al. Maternal obesity: a potential source of error in sonographic prenatal diagnosis. Obstet Gynecol 1990;76:339–42.

36. Hendler I, Blackwell SC, Treadwell MC, et al. Does advanced ultrasound equipment improve the adequacy of ultrasound visualization of fetal cardiac structures in the obese gravid woman? Am J Obstet Gynecol 2004;190:1616–9.

37. Maxwell C, Dunn E, Tomlinson G, et al. How does maternal obesity affect the routine fetal anatomic ultrasound? J Matern Fetal Neonatal Med 2010;23: 1187–92.

38. Dashe JS, McIntire DD, Twickler DM. Effect of maternal obesity on the ultrasound detection of anomalous fetuses. Obstet Gynecol 2009;113: 1001–7.

39. Nevo O, Frasca E, Toi A, et al. Transvaginal early anatomy ultrasound for obese women. Am J Obstet Gynecol 2011;204:S151.

40. Michailidis GD, Papageorgiou P, Economides DL. Assessment of fetal anatomy in the first trimester using two- and three-dimensional ultrasound. Br J Radiol 2002;75:215–9.

41. Fauchon DE, Benzie RJ, Wye DA, et al. What information on fetal anatomy can be provided by a single first-trimester transabdominal three-dimensional sweep? Ultrasound Obstet Gynecol 2008;31:266–70.

42. Bhaduri M, Fong K, Toi A, et al. Fetal anatomic survey using three-dimensional ultrasound in conjunction with first-trimester nuchal translucency screening. Prenat Diagn 2010;30:267–73.

43. Antsaklis A, Daskalakis G, Theodora M, et al. Assessment of nuchal translucency thickness and the fetal anatomy in the first trimester of pregnancy by two- and three-dimensional ultrasonography: a pilot study. J Perinat Med 2011;39:185–93.

44. Blumenfeld Z, Zimmer EZ, Weizman B, et al. The central nervous system. In: Bronshtein M, Zimmer EZ, editors. Transvaginal sonography of the normal and abnormal fetus. New York: The Parthenon publishing group; 2001. p. 41–64.

45. Nevo O, Bronshtein M. Fetal transient occipital bone protuberance during early pregnancy. Prenat Diagn 2010;30:879–81.

46. Moore KL, Persaud TV. The developing human - clinically oriented embryology. Philadelphia: Saunders; 2003. p. 329–464.

47. Mitchell SC, Korones SB, Berendes HW. Congenital heart disease in 56,109 births. Incidence and natural history. Circulation 1971;43:323–32.

48. Allan LD, Sharland G, Tynan MJ. The natural history of the hypoplastic left heart syndrome. Int J Cardiol 1989;25:341–3.

49. Paladini D, Calabro R, Palmieri S, et al. Prenatal diagnosis of congenital heart disease and fetal karyotyping. Obstet Gynecol 1993;81:679–82.

50. Bronshtein M, Zimmer EZ, Blazer S. Accuracy of transvaginal sonography for diagnosis of complete atrioventricular septal defect in early pregnancy. Am J Cardiol 2003;91:903–6.

51. Bronshtein M, Lorber A, Berant M, et al. Sonographic diagnosis of fetal vascular rings in early pregnancy. Am J Cardiol 1998;81:101–3.

52. Berg C, Kamil D, Geipel A, et al. Absence of ductus venosus-importance of umbilical venous drainage site. Ultrasound Obstet Gynecol 2006;28:275–81.

53. Camera G, Mastroiacovo P. Birth prevalence of skeletal dysplasias in the Italian Multicentric Monitoring System for Birth Defects. Prog Clin Biol Res 1982; 104:441–9.

54. Timor-Tritsch IE, Monteagudo A, Peisner DB. High-frequency transvaginal sonographic examination for the potential malformation assessment of the 9-week to 14-week fetus. J Clin Ultrasound 1992;20:231–8.

55. Zalen-Sprock RM, Brons JT, van Vugt JM, et al. Ultrasonographic and radiologic visualization of the developing embryonic skeleton. Ultrasound Obstet Gynecol 1997;9:392–7.

56. Chitty LS, Altman DG. Charts of fetal size: limb bones. BJOG 2002;109:919–29.

57. Rosati P, Guariglia L. Transvaginal fetal biometry in early pregnancy. Early Hum Dev 1997;49:91–6.

58. Zorzoli A, Kustermann A, Caravelli E, et al. Measurements of fetal limb bones in early pregnancy. Ultrasound Obstet Gynecol 1994;4:29–33.

59. Glanc P, Chitayat D. Prenatal diagnosis of the lethal skeletal dysplasias. Waltham (MA): Wolters Kluwer Health. Up to Date; 2011.

60. Chitty LS, Griffin DR. Prenatal diagnosis of fetal skeletal anomalies. Fetal Matern Med Rev 2008;19:135–64.

61. Khalil A, Pajkrt E, Chitty LS. Early prenatal diagnosis of skeletal anomalies. Prenat Diagn 2011;31:115–24.

62. Ngo C, Viot G, Aubry MC, et al. First-trimester ultrasound diagnosis of skeletal dysplasia associated with increased nuchal translucency thickness. Ultrasound Obstet Gynecol 2007;30:221–6.

63. Syngelaki A, Chelemen T, Dagklis T, et al. Challenges in the diagnosis of fetal non-chromosomal abnormalities at 11-13 weeks. Prenat Diagn 2011;31:90–102.

64. Krakow D, Alanay Y, Rimoin LP, et al. Evaluation of prenatal-onset osteochondrodysplasias by ultrasonography: a retrospective and prospective analysis. Am J Med Genet A 2008;146A:1917–24.

65. Superti-Furga A, Unger S. Nosology and classification of genetic skeletal disorders: 2006 revision. Am J Med Genet A 2007;143:1–18.

66. Doray B, Favre R, Viville B, et al. Prenatal sonographic diagnosis of skeletal dysplasias. A report of 47 cases. Ann Genet 2000;43:163–9.

67. Krakow D, Lachman RS, Rimoin DL. Guidelines for the prenatal diagnosis of fetal skeletal dysplasias. Genet Med 2009;11:127–33.

68. Schramm T, Gloning KP, Minderer S, et al. Prenatal sonographic diagnosis of skeletal dysplasias. Ultrasound Obstet Gynecol 2009;34:160–70.

69. Tretter AE, Saunders RC, Meyers CM, et al. Antenatal diagnosis of lethal skeletal dysplasias. Am J Med Genet 1998;75:518–22.

Demystifying Ovarian Cysts

Carrie B. Betel, MD*, Phyllis Glanc, MD, FRCPC (C)

KEYWORDS

- Ovary • Cyst • Ultrasound
- Imaging • Low malignant potential

Advances in ultrasonography, including higher-frequency probes and routine use of transvaginal ultrasonography, have led to increased detection of ovarian cystic lesions. Fortunately, these advances have also led to increased resolution, allowing characterization of approximately 90% of adnexal masses by ultrasonography alone.[1] In this article, the ultrasound technique and features of ovarian lesions as well as other imaging modalities in the armamentarium of ovarian lesion characterization are discussed. Various ovarian cystic lesions, including borderline tumors, are then evaluated. Clinical considerations and management are also discussed. This article is limited to intraovarian lesions. Extraovarian cystic lesions and lesions during pregnancy are not discussed, but the reader can refer to other articles for further information.[2,3]

IMAGING

Meticulous sonographic technique is essential when characterizing ovarian lesions. Transabdominal scanning provides a wider field of view for large lesions and can visualize ovaries that lie superior or lateral in the pelvis. However, transvaginal ultrasonography is the mainstay of evaluation. Any lesion must be visualized in its entirety in at least 2 planes. Ovarian tissue surrounding the lesion should be identified to confirm an ovarian origin.

Numerous studies have attempted to compile a list of sonographic criteria that can accurately predict malignancy, but none have sufficient specificity and sensitivity to rule in or rule out malignancy. There is simply too much overlap in appearance between benign and malignant lesions. Overall, a subjective pattern recognition approach has been shown to be better than scoring systems to characterize adnexal lesions, with a sensitivity of 88% to 100%, specificity of 62% to 96%, positive predictive value of 99%, and negative predictive value of 73%.[4–7]

Gray-scale morphology is the best determinant in evaluating if a lesion is benign or malignant.[8] Features suggestive of malignancy include thick and irregular walls or septations (>3 mm) and papillary projections (>3 mm).[4,9–13] However, mural or septal thickening can be seen in many benign conditions, such as endometriosis, abscess, and benign neoplasm.

Doppler ultrasonography can be qualitative or quantitative and is used as an adjunct to gray-scale ultrasonography. Qualitatively, malignancies display Doppler color flow centrally in solid components and septa because of neoangiogenesis; however, there is overlap with benign lesions.[14] A study by Stein and colleagues[7] looked at the presence of internal color flow in 170 adnexal masses and found a sensitivity of 77%, specificity of 69%, negative predictive value of 89%, and positive predictive value of 49%. Quantitatively, malignancies have a lower pulsatility index (PI), lower resistive index (RI), and higher velocity. This is due to a lower impedance related to neovascularity and abnormal arteriovenous shunts. Thresholds suggested to classify a mass as malignant include RI less than 0.4, PI less than 1.0, maximum velocity greater than 15 cm/s, and absent diastolic notch.[7,15] However, there is enough overlap that

The authors have nothing to disclose.

Department of Medical Imaging, University of Toronto, Sunnybrook Health Sciences Centre, 2075 Bayview Avenue, Toronto, ON M4N 3M5, Canada

* Corresponding author. Department of Medical Imaging, University of Toronto, Sunnybrook Health Sciences Centre, Room AG-280, 2075 Bayview Avenue, Toronto, ON M4N 3M5, Canada.

E-mail address: carrie.betel@sunnybrook.ca

Ultrasound Clin 7 (2012) 75–91

doi:10.1016/j.cult.2011.08.003

no definite numeric cutoff can be assigned.[7] For example, one study showed that 6 of 8 malignant lesions had an RI of greater than 0.4.[15] Malignancies can have a high PI or RI due to vascular tumor thrombi, vascular stenosis, aneurysmal dilatation, and abnormal vessel branching.

Ancillary sonographic features to suggest malignancy include involvement of adjacent pelvic organs and sidewalls, ascites, lymphadenopathy, and peritoneal, mesenteric, or omental nodularity.

There is little data regarding the role of 3-dimensional ultrasonography, but it may have value in determining lesion origin. Microbubble contrast ultrasonography may help detect neovascularity associated with early-stage ovarian cancer,[16] in which malignant ovarian masses have greater peak enhancement, longer washout time, and increased vascular volume.[17]

The sensitivity of computed tomography (CT) in detecting and characterizing adnexal masses is poorer than that of ultrasonography. CT has a sensitivity of 90%, specificity of 89%, positive predictive value of 78%, negative predictive value of 95%, and accuracy of 89%.[18] CT is superior to ultrasonography in assessing the extent of disease and detecting small peritoneal implants and lymphadenopathy. CT can also detect macroscopic fat, allowing for characterization of dermoids. Magnetic resonance (MR) imaging is a useful adjunct to ultrasonography because of its increased tissue specificity and larger field of view. MR imaging can characterize fat, blood, and simple fluid and demonstrate enhancement and thus be a problem-solving tool when ultrasonography is nondiagnostic. This technique can detect the ovary when not seen by ultrasonography, particularly in instances of distorted anatomy; this is helpful to determine the origin of a lesion. The sensitivity of MR imaging is 91% to 100%, and its specificity is 78% to 93%.[13,19]

Positron emission tomographic (PET) scan with fluorodeoxyglucose F 18 is not recommended for primary detection of ovarian cancer, with a sensitivity of 74% to 100% and specificity of 81% to 100%.[20,21] The technique's utility seems to lie in treatment planning, follow-up, and detection of recurrent disease.[13] False-negative results may be seen with borderline and low-grade malignancies, whereas false-positive results may be seen in hydrosalpinx, fibroids, and endometriomas.[13]

PHYSIOLOGIC CYSTS

Simple ovarian cysts are anechoic and thin walled, with distal acoustic enhancement and no solid component (Fig. 1). Typically, a single thin (<3 mm) septation would still permit the characterization of

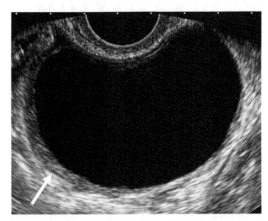

Fig. 1. Simple ovarian cyst in a 28-year-old woman. Arrow points to surrounding ovarian parenchyma, indicating an intraovarian location. No internal Doppler flow was seen (images not shown).

a cyst as simple and may be followed in a similar manner. Most simple cysts in premenopausal women are physiologic follicles. These cysts may enlarge up to 3 cm and generally resolve in 1 to 2 months.[14,22] Occasionally, they can hemorrhage, leading to a more complex appearance.[23] Some simple-appearing cysts are actually benign cystadenomas (especially those >10 cm and in older women).[24]

Numerous articles have been written about simple cysts in postmenopausal women. Initially such cysts were thought to be abnormal, but, as ultrasonography improves in resolution and these cysts are seen more frequently, their significance has been reevaluated. Currently, several studies have determined that simple cysts are seen in 10% to 20% of postmenopausal women and are unrelated to hormone replacement therapy or time since menopause.[25,26]

A study of 1769 asymptomatic postmenopausal women showed that 6.6% (116 women) had simple cysts smaller than 5 cm; of these, 24%[26] resolved, 59%[27] persisted, and 17%[18] were lost to follow-up.[28] Of the 27 that resolved, 56%[15] resolved in 6 months and the rest by 2 years. Of the persistent cysts, 26%[18] had surgery, and, of these, 67% were serous cystadenomas.[28]

Another study followed up 3259 simple unilocular cysts in 2763 women aged at least 50 years for a mean follow-up time of 6.3 years.[24] Of these, 69% (2261) resolved (66% within 3 months). There was no case of ovarian cancer developing from any of these cysts, and the investigators concluded that unilocular cysts have an extremely low risk of malignancy (<1% with 95% confidence interval).[24]

Corpora lutea are the remnants of a dominant follicle after ovulation.[22] They are unilateral and generally smaller than 3 cm.[14] Sonographic features include internal echoes, a thick crenulated wall, and peripheral vascularity (termed a ring of fire) (**Fig. 2**).[8,29–31] Internal hemorrhage can cause the size to increase to more than 5 cm.[32] These masses usually regress within 14 to 16 weeks of their formation.[23] Ideally, ultrasonography of premenopausal women should be performed on days 5 to 9 of the menstrual cycle (before ovulation) to minimize these findings.

POLYCYSTIC OVARIAN SYNDROME

Polycystic ovarian syndrome (PCOS) is an endocrine disorder diagnosed biochemically or by pathology. Sonographically, the ovary may be normal, but the diagnosis is suggested if the ovaries are enlarged and contain multiple small subcentimeter follicles.[33] One study looking at 28 patients between the ages of 17 and 39 years with biochemical evidence for PCOS showed the mean ovarian volume to be enlarged at 14 cm^3 (vs normal 9.8 cm^3); however, they were normal sized in 29.7% of women.[34] The ultrasonographic criteria for polycystic ovaries have evolved since the initial criteria reported in 1986. The 2003 Rotterdam criteria defined a polycystic ovary as the presence of 12 or more follicles that measure between 2 and 9 mm and/or increased ovarian volume (>10 mL).[35] A single ovary fitting this description permits the diagnosis of polycystic ovaries. Additional features reported variably include peripheral location of the follicles and hyperechoic central stroma. The most recent definition of PCOS published by the Androgen Excess and PCOS Society included hyperandrogenism (clinical or biochemical), ovarian dysfunction (oligoanovulation and/or polycystic ovaries), and the exclusion of related disorders.[36] Stein-Leventhal syndrome is an associated triad of amenorrhea, hirsutism, and obesity.[33] These patients are at risk for endometrial cancer due to increased estrogen levels. They also have an increased risk of ovarian tumors, with a frequency of 4.6% to 17.0%.[37]

OVARIAN HYPERSTIMULATION SYNDROME

Ovarian hyperstimulation syndrome is seen in patients receiving ovulation induction medications. This condition results in bilateral enlarged multicystic ovaries (**Fig. 3**) and can be associated with ascites and pleural effusion.[38]

HEMORRHAGIC CYST

Hemorrhage commonly occurs within a corpus luteum but occasionally occurs within a physiologic cyst.[14,22] Sonographic appearance is variable, depending on the age of the blood, and most show through transmission.[39,40] Internal echoes are usually seen; sometimes, sonographic gain must be increased to elicit subtle echoes.[40] Internal strands are often seen and are related to fibrin. Unlike septations, strands are numerous, thin, weak reflectors and do not traverse the entire cyst.[41] Their appearance has been described as fishnet, lacy, cobweb, or spiderweb.[14,22] An internal clot may mimic a solid component, but clots are avascular and have concave borders or angularity due to clot retraction (**Fig. 4**).[14] Blood clot may also show jellylike movement with transducer pressure.[4] Fluid-fluid levels,[42] peripheral vascular flow, and thick walls may be seen. Hemorrhagic cysts generally resolve within 8 weeks.[39] The importance of visualization of characteristic features of intralesional hemorrhage is that, virtually always, it represents a benign lesion. Although the hemorrhagic cyst has often been considered a challenging diagnosis, specific sonomorphologic features may permit specific diagnosis in as many as 90% of hemorrhagic cysts.[39,43]

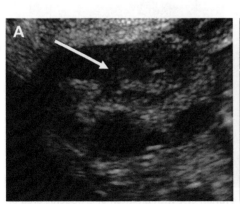
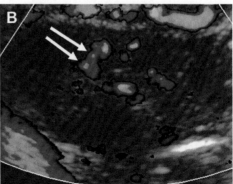

Fig. 2. Corpus luteum in a 28-year-old woman. Gray-scale image (*A*) shows a right ovarian cyst with internal echoes (*arrow*). Color Doppler image (*B*) shows a surrounding ring of fire (*double arrow*).

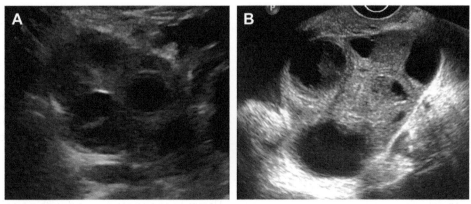

Fig. 3. Ovarian hyperstimulation syndrome in a 35-year-old woman. The right ovary (*A*) is imaged transabdominally, and the left ovary (*B*) is imaged transvaginally. Both ovaries contain multiple cysts.

ENDOMETRIOMA

Endometriosis is defined as the presence of functional endometrial tissue outside the uterus.[44] A focal cystic lesion is called an endometrioma. Incidence is 5% to 10% in women, predominantly in those of childbearing age.[44] Disease extent does not always correlate to symptom severity.[45] Multiplicity of lesions helps confirm the diagnosis, with the ovary being the most common site. Approximately 50% are bilateral.[45]

Sonographic appearance of an endometrioma is variable. Classically, a unilocular or multilocular cystic lesion is demonstrated with avascular homogeneous low-level internal echoes; this is seen in about 95% of endometriomas (**Fig. 5**).[46] Echogenic mural foci are seen in 36% of endometriomas, possibly mural cholesterol clefts (**Fig. 6**).[46] One study showed that the likelihood ratio of endometrioma is 5 in a cystic lesion with low-level echoes, increasing to 8 with absence of neoplastic features, and further increasing to 48 when there is multilocularity or echogenic mural foci.[46] Less typically, the cystic lesion may be anechoic, contain a fluid-fluid level or septation, or contain internal calcification.[47] A solid nodule is seen in 4% to 20% of endometriomas[46] representing blood clot or endometrial tissue (see **Fig. 5**B and C), and this can show Doppler flow if endometrial tissue is present within the nodule.[48] Real-time scanning with manual pressure can assess for secondary signs of adhesions, such as posterior displacement and fixed position of pelvic organs.[45]

The ultrasonographic appearance can overlap with hemorrhagic cyst, dermoid, or cystic neoplasm. Follow-up ultrasonography in premenopausal women in 6 to 12 weeks is helpful to distinguish from a hemorrhagic cyst.[22]

MR imaging can confirm the diagnosis because endometriotic deposits are bright on T1-weighted

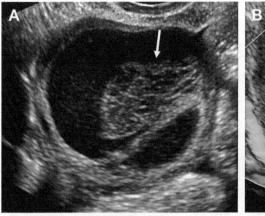
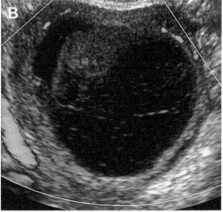

Fig. 4. Hemorrhagic cyst in a 33-year-old woman. Right ovarian cyst with an internal echogenic area on a grayscale image consistent with blood clot (*A*); arrow points to the concave margin, suggesting blood clot. Color Doppler image (*B*) shows no internal vascularity.

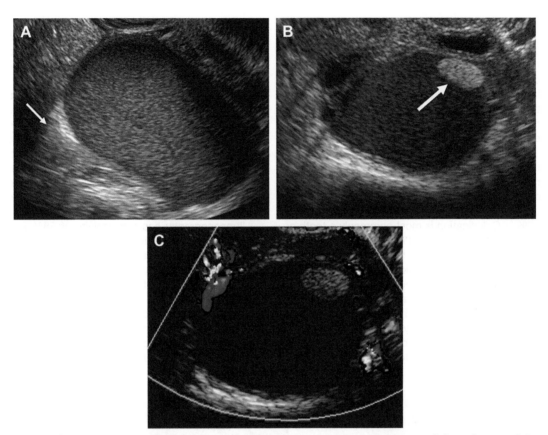

Fig. 5. Endometrioma in a 41-year-old woman (*A*) showing low-level internal echoes and through transmission (*arrow*). Endometrioma in a 28-year-old woman (*B*) showing low-level internal echoes and an echogenic mural nodule (*arrow*). Color Doppler image (*C*) shows no internal vascularity.

images (even with fat saturation) and dark on T2-weighted images (termed T2 shading).[22] MR imaging is superior in assessing disease extent due to the wider field of view and in detecting small endometriotic plaques. The sensitivity, specificity, and accuracy of MR imaging are 90%, 98%, and 96%, respectively.[49]

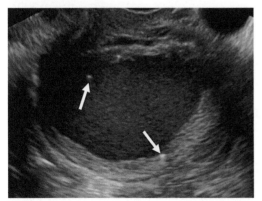

Fig. 6. Endometrioma in a 36-year-old woman. Endometrioma contains low-level echoes and echogenic mural foci (*arrows*).

Malignant transformation is rare, occurring in 0.6% to 0.8% of women with endometriosis.[50–52] The pathogenesis is unclear and may result from long-term exposure to unopposed estrogen.[13,50] The most common histologic types are endometrioid and clear cell carcinoma.[53] About 75% of cases are intraovarian.[50] These conditions are more likely to occur in women older than 45 years and in lesions larger than 9 cm.[54] Suspicion should be aroused when vascular mural nodules are seen or when there is rapid growth of a lesion.[55,56] MR imaging may show loss of T2 shading because of dilution of hemorrhagic fluid by tumor secretions.[55] Rarely during pregnancy, endometriomas may become decidualized, leading to development of vascular mural nodules that mimic the appearance of malignancy.[57] This decidualization is due to increased progesterone levels causing hypertrophy of endometrial stromal cells.

DERMOID

Dermoids, also termed mature cystic teratomas, are the most common benign ovarian tumor in young women and are often found incidentally.[58] These tumors comprise 20% of adult and 50% of pediatric ovarian tumors and 95% of germ cell tumors.[58,59] The other germ cell tumors are discussed later in this article. Although most common in women of reproductive age, these tumors can be seen in girls and postmenopausal women. Dermoids develop from mature tissues of ectodermal, endodermal, and mesodermal germ cell layers.

Sonographically, 88% of dermoids are a unilocular cyst, and 10% are bilateral.[60] The cystic lesion may contain fat, calcification, Rokitansky nodule, or dermoid mesh (**Fig. 7**A). Macroscopic fat is seen in 93% of dermoids and calcification in 56%.[58] Calcification is most commonly a tooth or bone; teeth are seen in 31% of cases.[60] Calcification is not highly specific because it can also be seen in malignancy. A Rokitansky nodule (or dermoid plug) is a mural nodule composed of fat, hair, sebaceous material, and calcification.[61] This nodule is often highly echogenic, with posterior acoustic shadowing.[62] Hyperechogenicity has a positive predictive value of 98% and is seen in 58% of teratomas.[62] Shadowing is due to internal

calcification, has a positive predictive value of 96%, and is seen in 86% of teratomas.[62] Dermoid mesh is seen as internal hyperechoic lines and dots; this feature has a positive predictive value of 98% and is seen in 61% of teratomas.[62] Fat-fluid levels with echogenic fat in a nondependent position were shown on ultrasonography to have a positive predictive value of 60% and are seen in 8% of teratomas (see **Fig. 7**B).[62,63] One case report describes multiple echogenic floating balls, which on pathology were desquamative keratin formations.[64] Hemorrhagic cysts may also be echogenic but do not display posterior acoustic shadowing.

Ultrasonography has a sensitivity of 58% and specificity of 99% in the diagnosis of dermoids.[65] CT can detect calcification, and fat within a cyst is diagnostic (see **Fig. 7**C). However, 15% of dermoids do not contain fat,[66] foci of fat may not be seen because of volume averaging with surrounding fat, and lipoleiomyomas also contain fat. On MR imaging, macroscopic internal fat is seen, which is bright on T1-weighted sequences with signal loss on fat saturation sequences.

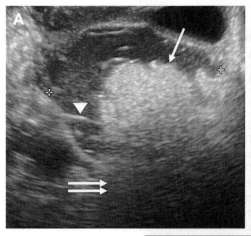
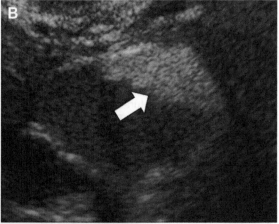
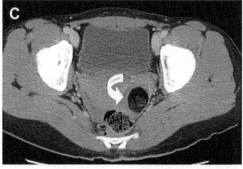

Fig. 7. Dermoid in the left ovary of a 28-year-old woman (*calipers*) showing many classic features (*A*). This includes an echogenic Rokitansky nodule (*arrow*), posterior shadowing (*double arrow*), and dermoid mesh (*arrowhead*). Dermoid in a 75-year-old woman (*B*) showing a fluid-fluid level (*large arrow*). (*C*) Contrast-enhanced CT scan in the same 75-year-old patient showing macroscopic fat within the dermoid (*curved arrow*).

Chemical shift artifact is seen in 62% to 87% of cases.[13] Dermoids are bilateral in 10%.[58,67]

Complications are rare and include rupture, torsion, malignant transformation, infection (1%), and autoimmune hemolytic anemia (<1%).[68] Rupture (1%–4%) with leakage of sebaceous fluid can cause inflammation.[27] Torsion (3%–16%) can cause engorged blood vessels and deviation of the uterus toward the torsion.[27] Malignant transformation is seen in 0.17% to 2.00%,[22] and more than 80% are squamous cell cancer.[27] The Rokitansky nodule is the most common site of transformation.[68] Features to suggest malignant transformation include postmenopausal women, size larger than 10 cm, solid component, central vascular flow, and extracapsular tumor growth.[68] Internal isoechoic branching structures have been described.[69] Generally, malignant transformation is an incidental microscopic focus, but occasionally local invasion and metastases can be seen.

OVARIAN TUMORS

The overall lifetime risk for a woman to be diagnosed with ovarian cancer is 1.8%.[70] Ovarian tumors are classified by the World Health Organization histologically as surface epithelial, germ cell, and sex cord–stromal tumors.[19] Metastases and other rare histologic conditions such as carcinosarcoma, primitive neuroendocrine tumor, and lymphoma also exist. Most germ cell and sex cord–stromal tumors are benign. Most tumors have a mixed cystic and solid appearance; however, some are predominantly solid, including Brenner, dysgerminoma, granulosa cell tumors, sex cord–stromal tumors, metastases, and lymphoma.

Epithelial Ovarian Tumors

Epithelial (or surface epithelial) ovarian tumors comprise 90% of ovarian cancers in the Western world[19] and are classified as serous (60%), mucinous (10%), endometrioid (15%), clear cell (5%), Brenner (also called transitional, 5%), mixed epithelial, and undifferentiated (8%) cancers.[16] The cell type of epithelial cancers may be benign, borderline, or malignant. Epithelial tumors peak in the sixth to seventh decade.[57] These tumors are predominantly cystic but often contain internal septa and nodules.

Serous tumors

Serous tumors are the most common benign and malignant ovarian neoplasm. They comprise 25% of benign ovarian neoplasms and up to 50% of ovarian cancers.[19] Of these, 60% are benign, 15% borderline, and 25% malignant.[23]

Serous cystadenomas are benign. They are well-defined large cystic lesions,[23] and 20% are bilateral.[71] These lesions are often unilocular with septations and papillary projections.[23]

Serous cystadenocarcinomas are malignant. These lesions too are cystic with septations and papillary projections but are often more complex in appearance than their benign counterparts (Fig. 8).[71] About 50% are bilateral.[71] More than 90% have an elevated cancer antigen 125 (CA 125) level.[19] Most patients present with advanced disease.[19]

Mucinous tumors

These tumors are less common than serous tumors. They comprise 20% of all ovarian tumors, 41% of benign ovarian neoplasms, and 10% of malignant ovarian tumors.[19,32] Of these, 80% are benign, 10% are borderline, and 5% are malignant.[23] These tumors are usually unilateral, only 2% to 5% are bilateral.[19]

Mucinous cystadenomas are large multiloculated cysts. Septations are smooth and thin. Internal locules may be echogenic on ultrasonography and hyperattenuating on CT.[71] On MR imaging, the locules are of varying signal intensity on T1- and T2-weighted images because of varying internal content of protein, mucin, and hemorrhage. This has been likened to a stained glass appearance.[72]

Mucinous cystadenocarcinoma has a similar appearance but with more papillary projections.[23] Overall, there are less solid components than serous tumors (Fig. 9).

Pseudomyxoma peritoneii occurs when these tumors metastasize or rupture and mucinous tumor implants develop on peritoneal surfaces. This condition is usually seen in borderline or malignant mucinous tumors.[73]

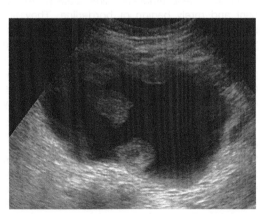

Fig. 8. Serous cystadenocarcinoma in a 56-year-old woman showing a right ovarian cyst with papillary projections by transabdominal imaging.

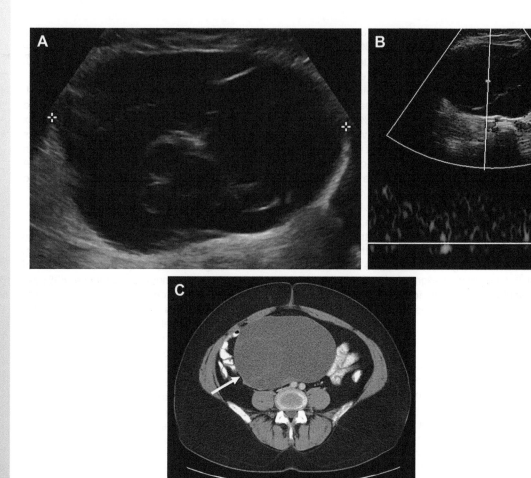

Fig. 9. Mucinous cystadenocarcinoma in a 41-year-old woman. The right ovary is replaced by a large cystic lesion with internal septations and locules (*A*). Color Doppler image shows arterial vascularity within a septation (*B*). Contrast-enhanced CT (*C*) of the same patient again shows a large cystic lesion with internal septations (*arrow*).

Endometrioid tumors

Endometrioid tumors comprise 17.5% of ovarian cancers.[19] These tumors are almost always malignant and rarely benign or borderline. They are bilateral in 25% of cases.[19] They may arise from the surface epithelium or endometriomas.[19] These tumors are associated with endometrial hyperplasia or cancer in 20% to 33% of cases.[74,75] Endometrioid tumors have a variable appearance and may be mixed cystic and solid or completely solid.

Clear cell tumors

Clear cell tumors comprise 7.4% of ovarian cancers.[19] These tumors are almost always malignant. About 75% present in stage 1 disease, and they have a good prognosis, with a 50% 5-year survival.[75] Clear cell tumors have a variable appearance, often a unilocular cyst with a mural nodule.[71]

Brenner tumors

Brenner tumors comprise less than 3% of epithelial ovarian neoplasms and are often discovered incidentally.[71] These tumors are rarely malignant and usually unilateral.[71] They are small, solid, well-defined tumors and may show extensive amorphous internal calcification.[76] In 20%, Brenner tumors are associated with ipsilateral mucinous cystic tumors, and, thus, imaging may show a solid and cystic appearance.[71] The internal fibrous stroma causes a low T2 signal on MR imaging.[19,76]

Other

Undifferentiated carcinoma shows cellular differentiation that is not sufficient to further characterize. These tumors are usually extensive at presentation with a poor prognosis.[71]

Cystadenofibromas are a subset of epithelial ovarian neoplasms that are usually benign.[32,77]

They are multiloculated cystic masses with septations and solid components (**Fig. 10**).[77] Nodules may be of low T2 signal on MR imaging because of a fibrous component.[77]

Germ Cell Tumors

Germ cell tumors include teratomas, dysgerminomas, choriocarcinomas, endodermal sinus tumors, embryonal carcinomas, and mixed germ cell tumors. Ovarian teratomas are further subdivided into mature teratomas, immature teratomas, and monodermal teratomas. Germ cell tumors comprise 15% to 20% of all ovarian neoplasms, but, of these, 95% are mature teratomas, which are discussed in the section "Dermoid."[23] Aside from teratomas, germ cell tumors are seen in children and young adults with a high frequency of malignancy.[23] Aside from mature teratomas, germ cell tumors are large predominantly solid masses that may show internal cystic components.[78] Some have elevated serum α-fetoprotein (AFP) and human chorionic gonadotropin (hCG) levels.[78]

Immature teratomas (also called malignant teratomas) comprise less than 1% of teratomas and are most commonly seen in adolescents and young women.[67] They are composed of immature or embryonic tissues, are malignant, and often present at an advanced stage with poor prognosis.[67] Half have an elevated AFP level.[78] These tumors are mostly solid with internal cystic areas and fat and are often quite large (12–25 cm) (**Fig. 11**).[60] Immature teratomas may contain calcification, which is cartilage or bone (as opposed to dermoids for which calcification is usually teeth). These tumors are associated with mature teratomas, which are seen in the same ovary in 26% and in the contralateral ovary in 10% of cases.[79] When treated with chemotherapy, immature teratomas can undergo maturation and appear similar to a mature teratoma, termed retroconversion.[80]

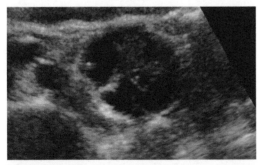

Fig. 10. Cystadenofibroma in a 71-year-old woman showing internal solid components within a cystic lesion.

Monodermal teratomas are teratomas with one tissue type predominating and include struma ovarii, ovarian carcinoid tumor, and tumor with neural differentiation.[67] Struma ovarii is a teratoma that predominantly contains thyroid tissue. Of these, 95% are benign and 5% show thyrotoxicosis.[68] The 5% that are malignant are most commonly papillary thyroid cancer, are generally large (>6 cm), and occur in older women.[81] Ovarian carcinoid tumor is seen as a solid mass and may be islet cell (insular), trabecular, or mucinous.[67] These tumors are seen in perimenopausal and postmenopausal women and are usually benign but have potential for malignancy (<2%). Carcinoid syndrome is uncommon.[58]

Other germ cell tumors are generally unilateral masses, predominantly solid with internal cystic or necrotic components. Dysgerminoma comprises less than 2% of ovarian cancers.[82] It is the most common malignant ovarian tumor in children, adolescents, and young adults, with 80% of patients presenting before 30 years of age.[19] Choriocarcinoma comprises less than 1% of ovarian tumors and is aggressive with an elevated serum hCG level.[58] This condition can be nongestational (primary) or gestational. Endodermal sinus tumor (also called yolk sac tumor) is a rare malignant germ cell tumor. It is aggressive with a poor prognosis and may have an elevated AFP level.[83]

Sex Cord–Stromal Tumors

Sex cord–stromal tumors are derived from sex cords and comprise 8% of ovarian neoplasms.[58] They include granulosa cell, fibroma, and Sertoli-Leydig tumors. Two-thirds of these tumors produce hormones, many with overt endocrine manifestations.[58] These manifestations include irregular menstrual cycles, menorrhagia, amenorrhea, and endometrial hyperplasia. Granulosa cell tumors and thecomas show hyperestrogenism, whereas Sertoli-Leydig tumors show hyperandrogenism.

Granulosa cell tumors are the most common malignant sex cord–stromal tumor, comprising 1% to 2% of all ovarian tumors[84] and 70% of all sex cord–stromal tumors.[58] There are adult type (95%) and juvenile tumors.[58,84] These tumors have a variable appearance, often multicystic septated masses, but they can be solid (**Fig. 12**).[84] More than 95% are unilateral.[58,84] Endometrial abnormalities such as hyperplasia are seen in 80% of cases because of estrogen production, with endometrial cancer in 10%.[85] These tumors have a good prognosis but can recur up to 25 years later.[86]

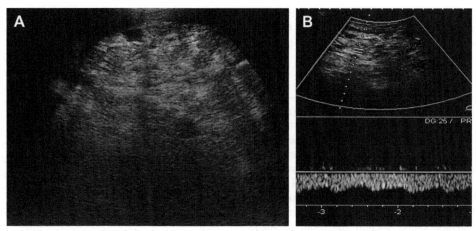

Fig. 11. Immature teratoma in a 28-year-old woman who was pregnant (22 weeks gestational age). The mass is echogenic and solid with small cystic areas (*A*). Color Doppler image shows internal arterial vascularity (*B*).

Fibromas, thecomas, and fibrothecomas are solid intraovarian masses arising from sex cord–stromal cells, are almost always benign, and comprise 4% to 5% of ovarian masses.[58,87] Fibromas are composed of fibroblasts and collagen, whereas thecomas are composed of theca cells, lipid, and fibrosis. Fibromas are often found incidentally in middle-aged women and are usually unilateral, although they may be bilateral in basal cell nevus syndrome.[58] Thecomas produce estrogen, which can lead to endometrial hyperplasia and cancer; however, this is less common than in granulosa cell tumors.[58] Sonographically, thecomas are solid ovarian masses with distal acoustic attenuation (**Figs. 13** and **14**).[58] They can have a small cystic component. Distal acoustic attenuation is seen in 18% to 52% of fibromas.[14] On MR imaging, thecomas are of homogeneous low signal on T1- and T2-weighted images with mild enhancement.[13] Meigs syndrome is seen in 1% of fibromas and is a triad of benign ovarian tumor (usually fibroma), ascites, and pleural effusion, which can mimic ovarian cancer but resolves on tumor resection.[58,88] Pseudo-Meigs syndrome is ascites and pleural effusion associated with mature teratoma, leiomyoma, cystadenoma, or ovarian malignancy.[58]

Sertoli-Leydig tumors comprise less than 1% of ovarian tumors.[58] They are the most common virilizing neoplasm.[58] Half are hormonally nonfunctional, 30% are virilizing, and a small amount are hyperestrogenic.[58] Three-fourths are less than 30 years old.[58] These tumors are often seen as unilateral solid small masses but may contain cysts. Only 1.5% are bilateral.[58] Sertoli-Leydig tumors are usually benign but may metastasize or recur after excision (20%).[58]

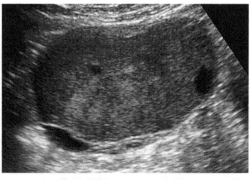

Fig. 12. Granulosa cell tumor in a 59-year-old woman. The mass is solid with small cystic areas. Internal vascularity was seen (image not shown).

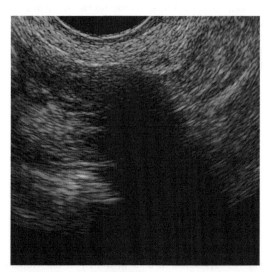

Fig. 13. Fibroma in the left ovary of a 46-year-old woman. Marked posterior shadowing is seen.

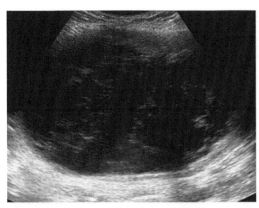

Fig. 14. Fibrothecoma in a 55-year-old woman is a partially cystic and solid mass with internal thick septations and solid nodules.

Tumors of Low Malignant Potential

Tumors of low malignant potential are also called borderline and atypical proliferative tumors and are malignant. These tumors comprise 15% to 20% of ovarian epithelial neoplasms, with an incidence of 1.5 to 2.5 per 100,000 women per year.[89,90] These tumors are usually seen in white women of reproductive age, slightly younger than women with malignant ovarian tumors.[90,91] Overall, a third of all ovarian malignancies in women younger than 40 years are borderline. In one study, the median age at diagnosis was 39 years, and 69% were younger than 45 years.[92] Symptoms are nonspecific, and 16% are asymptomatic at the time of diagnosis.[93] CA 125 levels may be marginally increased.[91]

Although these tumors are usually serous or mucinous, they can be endometrioid, clear cell, or Brenner tumors. In one study, 60% were serous, 37% mucinous, and 3% other (of which 4 of 10 were endometrioid).[92]

Histologically, there is cellular proliferation and moderate nuclear atypia, but the key to diagnosis is that there is no stromal invasion.[94]

Serous subtypes are the most common. These tumors are slow growing with peritoneal implants and regional lymphadenopathy. Histologically, 90% are typical and 10% are micropapillary.[90] One-third are bilateral. They are complex cystic masses with thin septations and solid components (**Fig. 15**).

Mucinous subtypes histologically are 90% intestinal and 10% müllerian.[90] Intestinal types are usually unilateral and, in 17% of cases, may coexist with pseudomyxoma peritoneii.[89] Müllerian types are bilateral in 40% and coexist with endometriomas in 20% to 30%.[89] They are unilocular or multilocular cystic masses with septations and solid components and may look like serous subtypes but are often much larger (**Fig. 16**).[90] The müllerian types have fewer locules.

Overall there is slightly less complexity than malignant ovarian masses and slightly more complexity than a cystadenoma.[91] Granberg and colleagues[95] showed that papillary projections are seen in 20% of benign, 62% of borderline, and 92% of malignant ovarian epithelial tumors, and the benign projections are smaller and less numerous. Ascites can be seen.[91]

CT and MR imaging may search for peritoneal implants. These tumors are not PET avid.[90]

These tumors are a subgroup of epithelial cancers with a more favorable prognosis. More than 75% are diagnosed at stage 1,[96] at which point the 5-year survival is more than 95%.[92] Of the serous subtype, at presentation, 70% are stage 1 confined to the ovary with 100% survival.[90] Of the mucinous subtype, 82% are confined to the ovary at presentation, with 99% to 100% survival, and 18% are of advanced stage, with 50% mortality.[90]

There is some uncertainty as to whether these tumors act as precursors to ovarian carcinoma. It has been postulated that these tumors are precursors to low-grade serous or mucinous ovarian cancers because both often share a common *KRAS* or *BRAF* mutation, whereas high-grade tumors usually arise de novo via a p53 mutation.[97,98] In a retrospective study, borderline and high-grade carcinoma pathologies with the same *KRAS* mutation coexisted in the same ovarian mass in 2 of 210 cases of serous carcinoma, suggesting a common precursor lesion.[97]

METASTASES

Ovarian metastases comprise 5% of ovarian tumors and 10% of ovarian cancers.[23] The 4 most common sites of origin are breast, lymph nodes, pelvis, and gastrointestinal tract (stomach, biliary, pancreas, colon).[23] Krukenberg tumors are ovarian metastases consisting of mucin-filled signet ring cells, typically gastric antral cancer, and also colon, appendix, breast, and, rarely, gallbladder, biliary, cervix, and bladder.[23]

These tumors are often bilateral.[23] They may be solid, partially cystic, or nearly completely cystic and may resemble primary ovarian cancers (**Fig. 17**). Lymphoma metastases are large, bilateral, and mostly solid without cystic areas or calcification (**Fig. 18**).

CLINICAL FACTORS

Risk factors for ovarian cancer relate to increased number of ovulations and include nulliparity, early

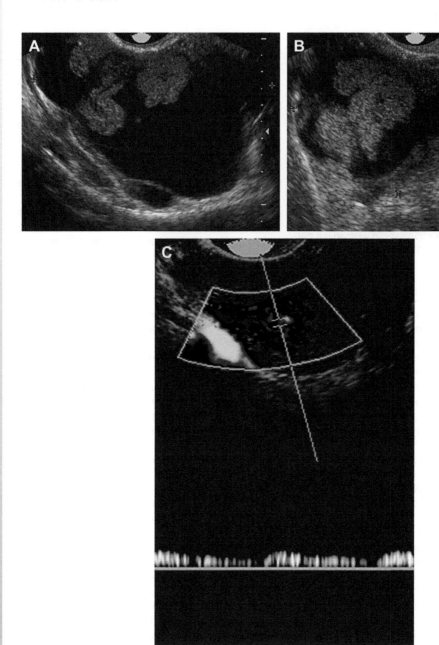

Fig. 15. Borderline serous tumor in a 23-year-old woman. Both the right (*A*) and left (*B*) ovaries have tumors that are cystic with internal solid components. Color Doppler image (*C*) shows arterial flow in the solid component of the right ovary (left lesion also showed flow, image not shown).

menarche, late menopause, age more than 50 years (postmenopausal), and gonadal dysgenesis.[71,99] Endometriosis increases the risk by up to 30%, possibly because of inflammation.[100] The use of oral contraceptive pills (OCP) decreases the risk, as does prior pregnancy and lactation.[100] There is a 30% to 40% decrease in risk with any prior OCP use and a 10% to 12% decrease with each year of use[100] This begins within a few months of use and can last more than 10 years after cessation.[101] Tubal ligation

decreases the risk by 40% to 70%, possibly because of decreased vascular supply to the ovary or blockage of retrograde menstruation, which causes inflammation.[100,102]

Less than 10% of ovarian cancers are associated with a known genetic mutation, usually *BRCA1* or *BRCA2*.[99] For women with these mutations, there is a life-time risk of 39% to 46% for *BRCA1* and 12% to 20% for *BRCA2*.[99] There is also an increased risk in patients with hereditary nonpolyposis colorectal cancer.[99]

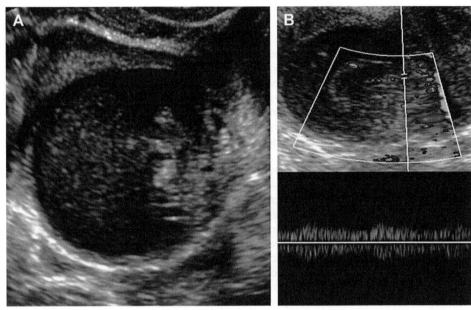

Fig. 16. Borderline mucinous tumor in a 38-year-old woman. Prior right borderline serous tumor resected 2 years previously (no images available). Left ovary contains a cystic lesion with an internal solid nodule (*A*). Color Doppler image shows arterial flow in the solid component (*B*).

Symptoms are nonspecific and can include abdominal and pelvic pain, distension, urinary frequency, early satiety, and constipation.[99]

CA 125 is a cancer antigen serum marker, elevated in about 80% of patients with ovarian cancer but only 50% of those with stage 1 disease.[32] It is present in 69% of mucinous tumors.[103] However, false-positive results are seen in benign conditions, particularly in premenopausal women, including pregnancy, endometriosis, fibroids, liver disease, benign ovarian cysts, and other malignancies (colon, uterine, fallopian tube, gastric, pancreatic).[16] Therefore, this marker is more useful in postmenopausal women and in monitoring disease response and recurrence posttreatment.

MANAGEMENT

When an ovarian cyst is not clearly characterized as either simple or benign etiology at the time of initial ultrasonography, several options are available, including short-term follow-up, MR imaging, or surgical consultation. Familiarity with the natural history and sonographic features of common ovarian cystic lesions helps to determine if a lesion can await spontaneous resolution or requires more immediate investigation.

The Society of Radiologists in Ultrasound recently published guidelines regarding the management of asymptomatic adnexal cysts in

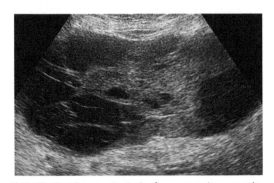

Fig. 17. Ovarian metastasis from a primary colon cancer in a 61-year-old woman.

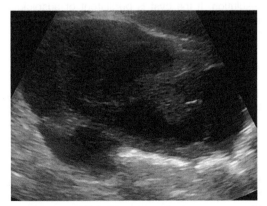

Fig. 18. Ovarian lymphoma metastasis in a 55-year-old woman.

nonpregnant women (both premenopausal and postmenopausal); the reader is referred to that article.[22]

In an attempt to decrease the number of follow-up studies, the investigators have recommended that a simple cyst smaller than 5 cm in a premenopausal woman requires no further follow-up. For a simple cyst between 5 and 7 cm, although almost certainly benign, annual follow-up was recommended. If a simple cyst larger than 7 cm was identified, MR imaging or surgical consultation was recommended; this recognizes the limitations of ultrasonography in characterizing a larger lesion.

In the postmenopausal population, because small simple cysts are very common, no follow-up is recommended in cysts that are 1 cm or smaller. In a cyst measuring 1 to 7 cm, annual follow-up was recommended to ensure stability, although they are almost certainly benign. As in the premenopausal patient, a cyst larger than 7 cm warrants further investigation with either MR imaging or surgical consultation. This investigation is also recommended when a cyst is not fully characterized with ultrasonography.

More than 70% of cysts in premenopausal women resolve over a 6-week period.[104] Also, 6 weeks ensure that the woman will be at a different stage in the menstrual cycle, preferably in the follicular phase (days 3–10).

If a complex cyst is confidently characterized as hemorrhagic, no follow-up is required unless they are larger than 5 cm, in which case short-term follow-up is appropriate, in 6 to 12 weeks. If a complex cyst is confidently characterized as an endometrioma, annual follow-up is recommended. A classic dermoid should have an initial 6- to 12-month follow-up to ensure stability.

Therefore, when unsure, a short-term follow-up is often the first step. If the cystic lesion is indeterminate but suggestive of a benign lesion, then a 6- to 12-month follow-up is performed to assess for resolution. If the cyst is persistent or suspicious in appearance, MR imaging and surgical consultation should be considered.

SUMMARY

Transvaginal ultrasonography is the primary imaging modality used to characterize ovarian cystic lesions and often the only modality required. This technique is all the more relevant because the incidence of identification of such lesions has risen so dramatically. A majority of these lesions are benign; however, it is important to identify lesions that are possibly malignant and to remember that some are low malignant potential tumors. Familiarity with the natural history of ovarian cystic lesions, characteristic imaging features, and published guidelines allows for a management approach for most encountered lesions. Clinical factors must be taken into account when assessing the patient. Taken together, this information can assist the physician interpreting the ultrasonography in demystifying the diagnosis and management of the unknown cystic ovarian lesion, which in turn provides a more focused differential diagnosis and more tailored management recommendations.

REFERENCES

1. Valentin L, Ameye L, Jurkovic D, et al. Which extrauterine pelvic masses are difficult to correctly classify as benign or malignant on the basis of ultrasound findings and is there is a way of making a correct diagnosis? Ultrasound Obstet Gynecol 2006;27(4):438–44.
2. Moyle PL, Kataoka MY, Nakai A, et al. Nonovarian cystic lesions of the pelvis. Radiographics 2010; 30(4):921–38.
3. Glanc P, Salem S, Farine D. Adnexal masses in the pregnant patient: a diagnostic and management challenge. Ultrasound Q 2008;24(4):225–40.
4. Valentin L. Use of morphology to characterize and manage common adnexal masses. Best Pract Res Clin Obstet Gynaecol 2004;18(1):71–89.
5. Timmerman D, Schwarzler P, Collins WP, et al. Subjective assessment of adnexal masses with the use of ultrasonography: an analysis of interobserver variability and experience. Ultrasound Obstet Gynecol 1999;13(1):11–6.
6. Van Calster B, Timmerman D, Bourne T, et al. Discrimination between benign and malignant adnexal masses by specialist ultrasound examination versus serum CA-125. J Natl Cancer Inst 2007; 99(22):1706–14.
7. Stein SM, Laifer-Narin S, Johnson MB, et al. Differentiation of benign and malignant adnexal masses: relative value of gray-scale, color Doppler, and spectral Doppler sonography. AJR Am J Roentgenol 1995;164(2):381–6.
8. Brown DL. A practical approach to the ultrasound characterization of adnexal masses. Ultrasound Q 2007;23(2):87–105.
9. Sassone AM, Timor-Trisch IE, Artner A, et al. Transvaginal sonographic characterization of ovarian disease: evaluation of a new scoring system to predict ovarian malignancy. Obstet Gynecol 1991;78(1):70–6.
10. Lerner JP, Timor-Tritsch IE, Federman A, et al. Transvaginal sonographic characterization of ovarian masses with an improved, weighted scoring system. Am J Obstet Gynecol 1994; 170(1Pt1):81–5.

11. Reles A, Wein U, Lichtenegger W. Transvaginal color Doppler sonography and conventional sonography in the preoperative assessment of adnexal masses. J Clin Ultrasound 1997;25(5):217–25.

12. Ferrazzi E, Zanetta G, Dordoni D, et al. Transvaginal ultrasonographic characterization of ovarian masses: comparison of five scoring systems in a multicenter study. Ultrasound Obstet Gynecol 1997;10(3):192–7.

13. Iyer VR, Lee SL. MRI, CT, and PET/CT for ovarian cancer detection and adnexal lesion characterization. AJR 2010;194(2):311–21.

14. Brown DL, Dudiak KM, Laing FC. Ultrasound characterization of adnexal masses. Radiology 2010;254(2):343–54.

15. Kurjak A, Zalud I, Alfirevic Z. Evaluation of adnexal masses with transvaginal color ultrasound. J Ultrasound Med 1991;10(6):295–9.

16. Dutta S, Wang F, Fleischer AC, et al. New frontiers for ovarian cancer risk evaluation: proteomics and contrast-enhanced ultrasound. AJR Am J Roentgenol 2010;194(2):349–54.

17. Fleischer AC, Lyshchik A, Andreotti RF, et al. Advances in sonographic detection of ovarian cancer: depiction of tumor neovascularity with microbubbles. AJR Am J Roentgenol 2010;194(2):343–8.

18. Tsili AC, Tsampoulas C, Charisiadi A, et al. Adnexal masses: accuracy of detection and differentiation with multidetector computed tomography. Gynecol Oncol 2008;110(1):22–31.

19. Imaoka I, Wada A, Kaji Y, et al. Developing an MR imaging strategy for diagnosis of ovarian masses. Radiographics 2006;26(5):1431–48.

20. Fenchel S, Grab D, Nuessle K, et al. Asymptomatic adnexal masses: correlation of FDG PET and histopathologic findings. Radiology 2002;223(3):780–8.

21. Rieber A, Nussle K, Stohr I, et al. Preoperative diagnosis of ovarian tumors with MR imaging: comparison with transvaginal sonography, positron emission tomography, and histologic findings. AJR 2001;177(1):123–9.

22. Levine D, Brown DL, Andreotti RF, et al. Management of asymptomatic ovarian and other adnexal cysts imaged at US: Society of Radiologists in Ultrasound consensus conference statement. Radiololgy 2010;256(3):943–54.

23. Sutton CL, McKinney CD, Jones JE, et al. Ovarian masses revisited: radiologic and pathologic correlation. Radiographics 1992;12(5):853–77.

24. Modesitt SC, Pavlik EJ, Ueland FR, et al. Risk of malignancy in unilocular ovarian cystic tumours less than 10 centimeters in diameter. Obstet Gynecol 2003;102(3):594–9.

25. Wolf SI, Gosink BB, Reldesman MR, et al. Prevalence of simple adnexal cysts in postmenopausal women. Radiology 1991;180(1):65–71.

26. Healy DL, Bell R, Robertson DM, et al. Ovarian status in healthy postmenopausal women. Menopause 2008;15(6):1109–14.

27. Comerci JT Jr, Licciardi F, Bergh PA, et al. Mature cystic teratoma: a clinicopathologic evaluation of 517 cases and review of the literature. Obstet Gynecol 1994;84(1):22–8.

28. Conway C, Zalud I, Dilena M, et al. Simple cyst in the postmenopausal patient: detection and management. J Ultrasound Med 1998;17(6):369–72.

29. Baerwald AR, Adams GP, Pierson RA. Form and function of the corpus luteum during the human menstrual cycle. Ultrasound Obstet Gynecol 2005;25(5):498–507.

30. Boune TH, Hagstrom H, Hahlin M, et al. Ultrasound studies of vascular and morphological changes in the human corpus luteum during the menstrual cycle. Fertil Steril 1996;65(4):753–8.

31. Sokalska A, Valentin L. Changes in ultrasound morphology of the uterus and ovaries during the menopausal transition and early postmenopausal: a 4-year longitudinal study. Ultrasound Obstet Gynecol 2008;31(2):210–7.

32. Jeong YY, Outwater EK, Kang HK. Imaging evaluation of ovarian masses. Radiographics 2000;20(2):1445–70.

33. Yeh H-C, Futterweit W, Thornton JC. Polycystic ovarian disease: US features in 104 patients. Radiology 1987;163(1):111–6.

34. Hann LE, Hall DA, McArdle CR, et al. Polycystic ovarian disease: sonographic spectrum. Radiology 1984;150(2):531–4.

35. Rotterdam ESHRE/ASRM-Sponsored PCOS Consensus Workshop Group. Revised 2003 consensus on diagnostic criteria and long-term health risks related to polycystic ovary syndrome. Hum Reprod 2004;19(1):41–7.

36. Assiz R, Carmina E, Dewailly D, et al. The Androgen Excess and PCOS Society criteria for the polycystic ovary syndrome: the complete task force report. Fertil Steril 2009;92(2):456–88.

37. Babaknia A, Calfopoulos P, Jones HW Jr. The Stein-Leventhal syndrome and coincidental ovarian tumors. Obstet Gynecol 1976;47(2):223–4.

38. McArdle CR, Sacks BA. Ovarian hyperstimulation syndrome. AJR Am J Roentgenol 1980;135(4):835–6.

39. Okai T, Kobayash K, Ryo E, et al. Transvaginal sonographic appearance of hemorrhagic functional ovarian cysts and their spontaneous regression. Int J Gynaecol Obstet 1994;44(1):47–52.

40. Baltarowich OH, Kurtz AB, Pasto ME, et al. The spectrum of sonographic findings in hemorrhagic ovarian cysts. AJR Am J Roentgenol 1987;148(5):901–5.

41. Patel MD. Practical approach to the adnexal mass. Radiol Clin North Am 2006;44(6):879–99.

42. Jain KA. Sonographic spectrum of hemorrhagic ovarian cysts. J Ultrasound Med 2002;21(8): 879–86.

43. Patel MD, Feldstein VA, Filly RA. The likelihood ratio of sonographic findings for the diagnosis of hemorrhagic ovarian cysts. J Ultrasound Med 2005;24: 607–14.

44. Olive DL, Schwartz LB. Endometriosis. N Engl J Med 1993;328(24):1759–69.

45. Woodward PJ, Sohaey R, Mezzetti TP Jr. Endometriosis: radiologic-pathologic correlation. Radiographics 2001;21(1):193–216.

46. Patel MD, Feldstein VA, Chen DC, et al. Endometriomas: diagnostic performance of US. Radiology 1999;210(3):739–45.

47. Bennett GL, Slywotzky CM, Cantera M, et al. Unusual manifestations and complications of endometriosis—spectrum of imaging findings: pictorial review. AJR Am J Roentgenol 2010;194(Suppl 6): WS34–46.

48. Guerriero S, Ajossa S, Mais V, et al. The diagnosis of endometriomas using colour Doppler energy imaging. Hum Reprod 1998;13(6):1691–5.

49. Togashi K, Nishimura K, Kimura I, et al. Endometrial cysts: diagnosis with MR imaging. Radiology 1991; 180(1):73–8.

50. Heaps JM, Nieberg RK, Berek JS. Malignant neoplasms arising in endometriosis. Obstet Gynecol 1990;75(6):1023–8.

51. Corner GW Jr, Hu C, Hertig AT. Ovarian carcinoma arising in endometriosis. Am J Obstet Gynecol 1950;59:760–76.

52. Scully RE, Richardson GS, Barlow JF. The development of malignancy in endometriosis. Clin Obstet Gynecol 1996;9(2):384–411.

53. Jimbo H, Yoshikawa H, Onda T, et al. Prevalence of ovarian endometriosis in epithelial ovarian cancer. Int J Gynaecol Obstet 1997;59(3):245–50.

54. Kobayashi H, Sumimoto K, Kitanaka T, et al. Ovarian endometrioma: risk factors of ovarian cancer development. Eur J Obstet Gynecol Reprod Biol 2008;138(2):187–93.

55. Tanaka YO, Yoshizako T, Nishida M, et al. Ovarian carcinoma in patients with endometriosis: MR imaging findings. AJR Am J Roentgenol 2000; 175(5):1423–30.

56. Wu TT, Coakley FV, Aqyyum A, et al. Magnetic resonance imaging of ovarian cancer arising in endometriomas. J Comput Assist Tomogr 2004;28(6): 836–8.

57. Machida S, Matsubara S, Ohawada M, et al. Decidualization of ovarian endometriosis during pregnancy mimicking malignancy: report of three cases with a literature review. Gynecol Obstet Invest 2008;66(4):241–7.

58. Shanbhogue AK, Shanbhogue DK, Prasad SR, et al. Clinical syndromes associated with ovarian neoplasms: a comprehensive review. Radiographics 2010;30(4):903–19.

59. Koonings PP, Campbell K, Mishell DR Jr, et al. Relative frequency of primary ovarian neoplasms: a 10-year review. Obstet Gynecol 1989;78(6): 921–6.

60. Caruso PA, Marsh MR, Minkowitz S, et al. An intense clinicopathologic study of 305 teratomas of the ovary. Cancer 1971;27(2):343–8.

61. Quinn SF, Erickson S, Black WC. Cystic ovarian teratomas: the sonographic appearance of the dermoid plug. Radiology 1985;155(2):477–8.

62. Patel MD, Feldstein VA, Lipson SD, et al. Cystic teratoma of the ovary: diagnostic value of sonography. AJR Am J Roentgenol 1998;171(4):1061–5.

63. Kim HC, Kim SH, Lee HJ, et al. Fluid-fluid levels in ovarian teratomas. Abdom Imaging 2002;27(1):100–5.

64. Kawamoto S, Sato K, Matsumoto H, et al. Multiple mobile spherules in mature cystic teratoma of the ovary. AJR Am J Roentgenol 2001;176(6):1455–7.

65. Mais V, Guerriero S, Ajossa S, et al. Transvaginal ultrasonography in the diagnosis of cystic teratoma. Obstet Gynecol 1995;85(1):48–52.

66. Yamashita Y, Hatanaka Y, Torashima M, et al. Mature cystic teratomas of the ovary without fat in the cystic cavity: MR features in 12 cases. AJR Am J Roentgenol 1994;163(3):613–6.

67. Outwater EK, Siegelman ES, Hunt JL. Ovarian teratomas: tumor types and imaging characteristics. Radiographics 2001;21(2):475–90.

68. Park SB, Kim JK, Kim KR, et al. Imaging findings of complications and unusual manifestations of ovarian teratomas. Radiographics 2008;28(4): 969–83.

69. Mlikotic A, McPhaul L, Hansen GC, et al. Significance of the solid component in predicting malignancy in ovarian cystic teratomas: diagnostic considerations. J Ultrasound Med 2001;20(8):859–66.

70. Jemal A, Siegel R, Ward E, et al. Cancer statistics 2009. CA Cancer J Clin 2009;59(4):225–49.

71. Wagner BJ, Buck JL, Seidman JD, et al. Ovarian epithelial neoplasms: radiologic-pathologic correlation. Radiographics 1994;14(6):1351–74.

72. Tanaka YO, Nishida M, Kurosaki Y, et al. Differential diagnosis of gynaecological "stained glass" tumours on MRI. Br J Radiol 1999;72(856):414–20.

73. Prayson RA, Hart WR, Petras RE. Pseudomyxoma peritonei: a clinicopathologic study of 19 cases with emphasis on site of origin and nature of associated ovarian tumors. Am J Surg Pathol 1994; 18(6):591–603.

74. Young RH, Scully RE. Pathology of epithelial tumors. Hematol Oncol Clin North Am 1992;6(4): 739–59.

75. Tornos C, Silva EG. Pathology of epithelial ovarian cancer. Obstet Gynecol Clin North Am 1994; 21(1):63–77.

76. Moon WJ, Koh BH, Kim SK, et al. Brenner tumor of the ovary: CT and MR findings. J Comput Assist Tomogr 2000;24(1):72–6.

77. Outwater IK, Siegelman ES, Talerman A, et al. Ovarian fibromas and cystadenofibromas: MRI features of the fibrous component. J Magn Reson Imaging 1997;7(3):465–71.

78. Brammer HM, Buck JL, Hayes WS, et al. Malignant germ cell tumors of the ovary: radiologic-pathologic correlation. Radiographics 1990;10(4):715–24.

79. Yanai-Inbar I, Scully RE. Relation of ovarian dermoid cysts and immature teratomas: an analysis of 350 cases of immature teratomas and 10 cases of dermoid cyst with microscopic foci of immature tissue. Int J Gynecol Pathol 1987;6(3):203–12.

80. Moskovic E, Jobling T, Fisher C, et al. Retroconversion of immature teratoma of the ovary: CT appearances. Clin Radiol 1991;43:402–8.

81. Caspi B, Appelman Z, Rabinerson D, et al. The growth pattern of ovarian dermoid cysts: a prospective study in premenopausal and postmenopausal women. Fertil Steril 1997;68(3):501–5.

82. Ulbright TM. Germ cell tumors of the gonads: a selective review emphasizing problems in differential diagnosis, newly appreciated, and controversial issues. Mod Pathol 2005;18(2 Suppl 2):S61–79.

83. Kurman RJ, Norris HJ. Endodermal sinus tumor of the ovary: a clinical and pathologic analysis of 71 cases. Cancer 1976;38(6):2404–19.

84. Ko SF, Wan YL, Ng SH, et al. Adult ovarian granulosa cell tumors: spectrum of sonographic and CT findings with pathologic correlation. AJR Am J Roentgenol 1999;172(5):1227–33.

85. Schumer ST, Cannistra SA. Granulosa cell tumor of the ovary. J Clin Oncol 2003;21(6):1180–9.

86. Hasiakos D, Papakonstantinou K, Karvouni E, et al. Recurrence of granulosa cell tumor 25 years after initial diagnosis: report of a case and review of the literature. Eur J Gynaecol Oncol 2008;29(1):86–8.

87. Bazot M, Ghossain MA, Buy JN, et al. Fibrothecomas of the ovary: CT and US findings. J Comput Assist Tomogr 1993;17(5):754–9.

88. Meigs JV, Cass JW. Fibroma of the ovary with ascites and hydrothorax: with a report of seven cases. Am J Obstet Gynecol 1937;33:249–67.

89. Acs G. Serous and mucinous borderline (low malignant potential) tumors of the ovary. Am J Clin Pathol 2005;123(Suppl):S13–57.

90. Lalwani N, Shanbhogue AK, Vikram R, et al. Current update on borderline ovarian neoplasms. AJR Am J Roentgenol 2010;194(2):330–6.

91. deSouza NM, O'Neill RO, McIndoe GA, et al. Borderline tumors of the ovary: CT and MRI features and tumor markers in differentiation from stage 1 disease. AJR Am J Roentgenol 2005;184(3):999–1003.

92. Zanetta G, Rota S, Chiari S, et al. Behavior of borderline tumors with particular interest to persistence, recurrence, and progression to invasive carcinoma: a prospective study. J Clin Oncol 2001;19(10):2658–64.

93. Webb PM, Purdie DM, Grover S, et al. Symptoms and diagnosis of borderline, early and advanced epithelial ovarian cancer. Gynecol Oncol 2004;92(1):232–9.

94. Stalsberg H, Abeler V, Blom P, et al. Observer variation in histologic classification of malignant and borderline ovarian tumors. Hum Pathol 1988;19(9):1030–5.

95. Granberg S, Wikland M, Jansson I. Macroscopic characterization of ovarian tumors and the relation to the histological diagnosis: criteria to be used for ultrasound evaluation. Gynecol Oncol 1989;35(2):139–44.

96. Barakat RR. Borderline tumors of the ovary. Obstet Gynecol Clin North Am 1994;21(1):93–105.

97. Dehari R, Kurman RJ, Logani S, et al. The development of high-grade serous carcinoma form atypical proliferative (borderline) serous tumors and low-grade micropapillary serous carcinoma. Am J Surg Pathol 2007;31(7):1007–12.

98. Lalwani N, Prasad SR, Vikram R, et al. Histologic, molecular, and cytogenetic features of ovarian cancers: implications for diagnosis and treatment. Radiographics 2011;31(3):625–46.

99. Stany MP, Maxwell GL, Rose GS. Clinical decision making using ovarian cancer risk assessment. AJR Am J Roentgenol 2010;194(2):337–42.

100. Modugno F, Ness RB, Allen GO, et al. Oral contraceptive use, reproductive history, and risk of epithelial ovarian cancer in women with and without endometriosis. Am J Obstet Gynecol 2004;191(3):733–40.

101. Daly MB. The epidemiology of ovarian cancer. Hematol Oncol Clin North Am 1992;6(4):729–38.

102. Riman T, Dickman PW, Nilsson S, et al. Risk factors for invasive epithelial ovarian cancer: results from a Swedish case-control study. Am J Epidemiol 2002;156(4):363–73.

103. Hempling RE. Tumor markers in epithelial ovarian cancer: clinical applications. Obstet Gynecol Clin North Am 1994;21(1):41–61.

104. Spanos WJ. Preoperative hormonal therapy of cystic adnexal masses. Am J Obstet Gynecol 1973;116(4):551–6.

Sonographic Depiction of Ovarian and Uterine Vasculature: New Techniques and Clinical Applications

Maria Piraner, MD[a], Arthur C. Fleischer, MD[b,c],*,
Andrej Lyshchik, MD, PhD[d], Rochelle F. Andreotti, MD[c,e]

KEYWORDS

- Color Doppler sonography • 3D pelvic sonography
- Ovarian vascularity contrast-enhanced ovarian sonography
- Uterine vascularity • Adnexal mass evaluation
- Adnexal torsion • Macrovascularity • Microvascularity

Transvaginal gray-scale imaging provides morphologic evaluation of the uterus and ovary, including assessment of internal structures such as septae, papillary excrescences, and wall structures. Color Doppler sonography and spectral analysis are used to depict their vascularity (**Fig. 1**). Three-dimensional (3D) (volumetric) sonography is often used to provide detailed assessment in addition to that obtained with two-dimensional (2D) imaging, showing spatial relationships and vascular morphology. 3D sonography can depict uterine and ovarian neovascularity and show aberrant vessel clusters, branching, and irregular caliber, which are seen in tumors within the pelvic organs.[1]

Qualitative and quantitative assessment of sonographically derived volume data is now available on most advanced scanners (**Box 1**). Quantitatively, virtual organ computer-aided analysis (VOCAL) offers a reliable, practical, noninvasive method to calculate indices of vascularity.[2] Tomographic ultrasound imaging (TUI) is a method by which multiple thin-sliced planar sections within a volume are displayed, bringing sonography closer to other forms of cross-sectional imaging such as computed tomography (CT). The high

Some of the data cited were obtained from studies supported by NIH/NCI grant R21 CA125227-01 and AIUM seed grants in 2001, 2003, 2009. The authors have nothing else to disclose.

[a] Women's Imaging, Department of Radiology and Radiological Sciences, Vanderbilt University Medical Center, CCC-1121 MCN, 1161 21st Avenue South, Nashville, TN 37232-2675, USA
[b] Department of Radiology and Radiological Sciences, Vanderbilt University Medical Center, RR-1213 MCN, 1161 21st Avenue South, Nashville, TN 37232-2675, USA
[c] Department of Obstetrics and Gynecology, Vanderbilt University Medical Center, Nashville, TN, USA
[d] Interventional Radiology, Department of Radiology and Radiological Sciences, Vanderbilt University Medical Center, CCC-1121 MCN, 1161 21st Avenue South, Nashville, TN 37232-2675, USA
[e] Department of Radiology and Radiological Sciences, Vanderbilt University Medical Center, CCC-1121 MCN, 1161 21st Avenue South, Nashville, TN 37232-2675, USA
* Corresponding author. Department of Radiology and Radiological Sciences, Vanderbilt University Medical Center, RR-1213 MCN, 1161 21st Avenue South, Nashville, TN 37232-2675.
E-mail address: arthur.fleischer@vanderbilt.edu

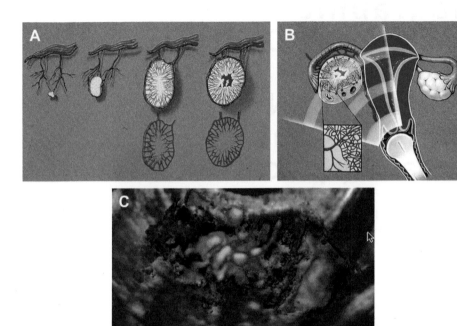

Fig. 1. Tumor vascularity with color Doppler sonography. (*A*) Tumor neoangiogenesis involves induction of vessels from host vasculature. The vascular network is irregular and focal areas of ischemia develop internally as the tumor grows from a few millimeters to a few centimeters (*left* to *right*). (*B*) Transvaginal color Doppler sonography can depict vessel density and branching of the macroscopic vessels. Contrast-enhanced transvaginal sonography (CE-TVS) is required to depict microvascularity. (*C*) Three-dimensional (3D) transvaginal (TV) color Doppler sonography of functioning corpus luteum showing peripheral vessels.

resolution, lack of ionizing radiation, and cost of sonography make it the diagnostic modality of choice for evaluation of pelvic disorders.

Contrast-enhanced transvaginal sonography (CE-TVS) is used for detection of ovarian cancer and certain fertility disorders. It can depict both macrovascularity (arteries, arterioles, veins, venules) and microvascularity (capillaries).[3,4] With addition of 3D and CE-TVS, overall ovarian, uterine, and endometrial perfusion can be shown (**Box 2**). By quantifying the signal intensity/time curves after the injection of the microbubbles, tumors have been shown to exhibit significantly different enhancement patterns compared with normal tissues.[3–6] These techniques have the potential to assess response of the ovary and endometrium to various treatment regimens. In oncology, this technique might be used for pretreatment and posttreatment assessment of the potential tumor response.[7]

Box 1
Vascular predictors of malignancy with 3D color Doppler sonography

Qualitative

- Central location
- Vessel clusters
- Abnormal branching
- Variable vessel caliber

Quantitative

- Increased vascularization index (VI), flow index (FI), vascular flow index (VFI)
- Increased fractal dimension

Box 2
Prediction of ovarian cancer with CE-TVS

Quantitative

- High peak enhancement (in dB)
- Long washout (in seconds)
- High area under the curve (AUC) (in seconds^{-1})

Qualitative

- High vessel density
- Vessel clusters in morphologically abnormal areas

This article reviews some of the new techniques for sonographic imaging of the ovaries and uterus, including color Doppler sonography, 3D sonography, and CE-TVS. Clinical applications and proposed areas for future research are discussed.

NEW TECHNIQUES/INSTRUMENTATION

3D sonography is used to provide a more detailed morphologic assessment than 2D sonography and to show spatial relationship and vascular morphology (**Figs. 2–4**).[1] Qualitative and quantitative assessment of volumetric data are obtained. 3D sonography is superior to 2D sonography in evaluation of papillary projections, showing characteristics of cyst walls, identifying extent of capsular infiltration of tumors, calculating ovarian volume, and showing the location of masses in relation to normal ovarian tissues (**Fig. 5**).[1,8]

3D sonography is also helpful in assessing tumor vascularity and angiogenesis.[1] 3D volume acquisition allows accurate volume measurements

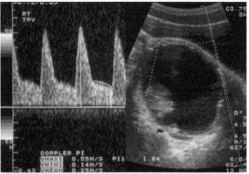

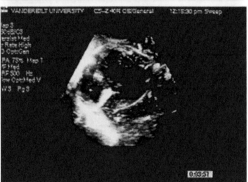

Fig. 3. 2D transabdominal (TA) color Doppler sonography (*top*) and 3D color Doppler sonography (*bottom*) of a papillary cystadenocarcinoma showing a large vessel within a mural nodule.

of regions within the volume and their relative vascularity. As opposed to 2D assessments of volume, it has been shown that volumetric measurements performed on a 3D sonography data set are more reliable.[2] In addition, the relative distribution of internal vascularity (central, peripheral, mixed) can be determined. Improvements in computer software allow VI, FI, and VFI to be quantified, allowing an objective assessment of vascularity with 3D color Doppler sonography (**Boxes 3–5**). The VI represents the amount of color signal detected in region of interest. FI represents the intensity of color signal in the region of interest. VFI represents the amount of color signal and its intensity within a region of interest. Studies have shown excellent intraobserver and interobserver reliability of VI, FI, and VFI, supporting the role of 3D power Doppler sonography as a method for assessing the physiologic function of the ovary and uterus.[2,9]

Contrast-enhanced sonography can be an adjunct to morphologic assessment with 2D and 3D and has been shown to be useful for early detection of ovarian cancer.[3] It also provides a means for evaluation of uterine and ovarian vascularity in a variety of conditions.[4–6] As in other

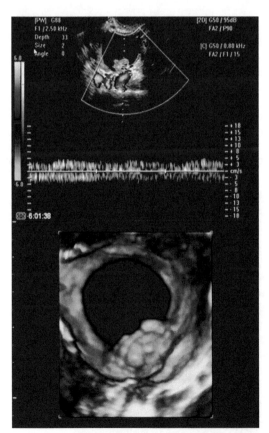

Fig. 2. 2D TV color Doppler (*top*) and 3D transvaginal sonography (TVS) (*bottom*) of a papillary cystadenoma showing abnormal vessels with low-impedance flow within the papillary excrescences.

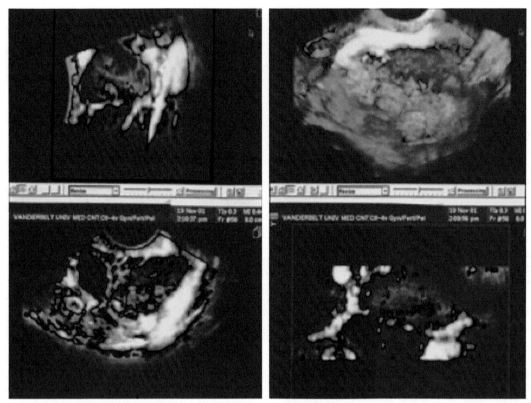

Fig. 4. Multiplanar reconstruction (first image, long axis; second image, coronal; third image, short axis) and fused 3D gray-scale and color Doppler sonography (fourth image) of an ovarian cancer showing abnormally branching vessels within a focally thickened area.

organs of the body, such as the liver, contrast-enhanced sonography has been shown to provide important information concerning the probability of malignancy in morphologically equivocal ovarian masses (**Fig. 6**).[3,4] Microbubble enhancement affords the direct depiction of tumor neovascularity, as shown by clustered vessels of irregular caliber and arrangement. By quantifying signal

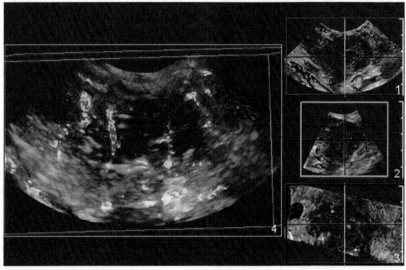

Fig. 5. 3D TV color Doppler sonography of normal ovary in a premenopausal woman showing regularly spaced vessels surrounding a functioning corpus luteum.

Box 3
Definition of VI

$$VI = \frac{C}{E}$$

GI 3DQ $\dfrac{\text{No. of color voxels}}{(\text{Total voxels} - \text{Background voxels})}$

ROI $\dfrac{\text{No. of color pixels}}{(\text{Total pixels} - \text{Background pixels})}$

Represents amount of color signal detected in region of interest.

Box 5
Definition of VFI

$$VFI = \frac{\sum_{c=1}^{c} Ic}{E}$$

GI 3DQ $\dfrac{\text{Amplitude} - \text{weighted color voxels}}{(\text{Total voxels} - \text{Background voxels})}$

ROI $\dfrac{\text{Amplitude} - \text{weighted color pixels}}{(\text{Total voxels} - \text{Background pixels})}$

Represents both the amount of color signal and its intensity within a region of interest.

---

intensity (in decibels)/time (seconds) curves after the injection of the microbubbles, tumors can be shown to exhibit significantly different enhancement compared with normal tissues (see **Fig. 6**). The microvascularity can be assessed using microbubble contrast, which depicts microvascularity better than color Doppler techniques. This difference is caused by the lack of blooming and poor temporal resolution inherent in color Doppler techniques compared with pulse inversion harmonic imaging.

Initial reports using contrast enhancement and color Doppler sonography showed that both the baseline and maximum Doppler intensities and their absolute and relative increases were significantly higher in malignancies (**Fig. 7**).[4] In addition, the arrival times were shorter and total duration of contrast (AUC) was longer in malignancies.[5,6] Tumors also have significantly greater vascular volume, as depicted by differences in the AUC.

Contrast-enhanced sonography using microbubbles has the potential to provide a means to assess tumor response to various therapeutic regimens, particularly in the light of the increased potential use of antiangiogenic agents and the importance of monitoring tumor response.[7] Labeled microbubbles to vascular endothelial growth factor (VEGF) receptors have shown promise in detecting areas of tumor growth. Other potential clinical uses of CE-TVS include assessment of ovulation disorders, ovarian hyperstimulation, and adnexal torsion, in which there are various degrees of vascular impairment, ischemia, or necrosis.

OVARIAN MASSES

A reliable preoperative determination between benign and malignant lesions contributes to

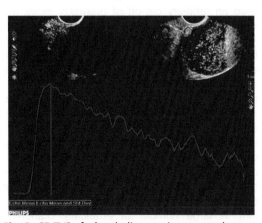

Fig. 6. CE-TVS of a borderline mucinous cystadenocarcinoma. The top right image shows an enhancing papillary excrescence. Region of interest is outlined in red. TV- color Doppler sonography (*top right image*) shows internal echogenic material thought to represent mucin. The time intensity curve (*bottom*) shows high peak intensity (20 dB) and slow washout time (161 seconds), which indicates tumor neovascularity.

Box 4
Definition of FI

$$FI = \frac{\sum_{c=1}^{c} Ic}{C}$$

GI 3DQ $\dfrac{\text{Amplitude} - \text{weighted color voxels}}{\text{Color voxels}}$

ROI $\dfrac{\text{Amplitude} - \text{weighted color pixels}}{\text{Color pixels}}$

Represents intensity of color signal in region of interest.

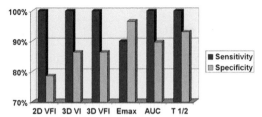

Fig. 7. Bar graphs showing sensitivity and specificity of 2D VFI and 3D VI, 3D VFI versus contrast-enhanced (CE) parameters including peak enhancement (Emax), AUC, and washout time ($T_{1/2}$). Of all parameters, AUC had the best sensitivity and specificity. Overall, CE-TVS had better sensitivity and specificity than 2D and 3D TVS color Doppler sonography.

improved management of patients with adnexal masses. Patients with benign masses may be observed or treated with laparoscopy and have a shorter hospital stay and lower morbidity compared with patients having laparotomy and more extensive surgeries required for malignancies. In addition, sonography provides important information regarding the proper surgical approach and postoperative management of lesions suspected to be malignant.

Transvaginal 2D gray-scale imaging provides morphologic information and orientation of pelvic structures and is essential before advanced imaging techniques in ultrasound. Color and power Doppler sonography, as well as spectral analysis, are used to evaluate the vascularity of pelvic structures.

In preliminary studies, some investigators have used an arbitrary cut-off of pulsatility index (PI) less than 1.0 or resistive index (RI) less than 0.4 as an indication of malignancies.[10,11] However, the accuracy of these cut-off values depends on which vessels were sampled. These indices should be interpreted in the context of morphologic and clinical findings. Low-resistance flow and the presence of centrally located vessels in an area suggest malignancy; however, these findings can be seen in some inflammatory conditions, decidualized endometriomas, and endocrinologically active tumors, as well as normal postovulatory ovaries. Therefore, correlations of the sonographic and clinical findings remain important. A large number of erratically branching vessels with changes in caliber, and centrally located flow within an ovarian mass, regardless of the RI or PI, should be taken as strongly suggesting malignancy.

It has been shown that 3D is superior to 2D imaging in distinguishing benign versus malignant masses by improved evaluation of papillary projections, showing characteristics of cyst walls,

identifying the extent of capsular infiltration of tumors, and detection of irregular internal and external mural nodules. Sonographic evaluation in 3D can estimate the amount of tumor relative to normal remaining ovarian tissues (see **Fig. 5**).[12]

3D sonography with power Doppler is useful in the evaluation of morphologically indeterminate adnexal masses. In particular, sonographic detection of central vascular flow, flow in excrescences, or irregular septations, and chaotic or complex architecture of vascularity suggest malignancy (**Figs. 2–5**). 3D color Doppler sonography can depict the vessel caliber and branching within an ovarian mass (**Fig. 8**; see **Box 1**). Ovarian tumors tend to have vessels that have abnormal caliber, with areas of stenosis and aneurysmal dilatation, as well as irregular branching. These features of the macroscopic smaller vessels can be seen using 3D color Doppler sonography.

The color mapping of the vascular architecture with 3D color Doppler sonography revealing location of vessels within the lesion is of particular importance. The presence of central intratumoral

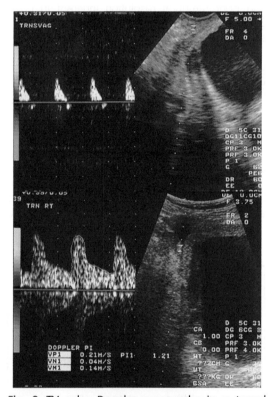

Fig. 8. TV color Doppler sonography in a torsed hemorrhagic ovary showing absent diastolic flow in the adnexal branch of the uterine artery (*top*) and intermediate impedance flow near the ovary (*bottom*). At surgery, a torsed hemorrhagic cyst was found.

vascularity was reported by Fleischer and colleagues[1] to have a 90% positive predictive value for predicting malignancy. In contrast, the absence of such central vascularity had a high negative predictive value of 96%. In another study involving 181 women with 144 benign, 11 borderline, and 26 malignant masses, Geomini and colleagues[13] reported significant differences in the incidence of central vessels in benign (15%) versus borderline (27%) and malignant (69%) adnexal masses, concluding that data acquired by 3D sonography and 3D power Doppler sonography could aid in differentiation between benign and malignant ovarian masses. The addition of 3D sonography to 2D power Doppler sonography was found to increase accuracy in detecting malignant adnexal masses where the solid portion of the mass was greater than 10 mL.[14]

In a European multicenter study that described guidelines for discrimination between benign and malignant adnexal masses based on multiple parameters using gray-scale and color Doppler sonography, certain rules were derived.[15] Evaluation of blood flow in papillary projections was performed with Doppler parameters involving RI, PI, peak systolic velocity, and time-averaged maximum velocity (TAMX), as well as estimation of color score ranging from no flow (score 1) to high flow (score 4). The masses with high values (score 4) were more likely to be malignant than those that were hypovascular.[15,16]

Data obtained from 30 benign and 8 malignant ovarian masses evaluated with 2D color Doppler sonography by Wilson and colleagues[16] showed a significant difference in VI and FI in benign versus malignant masses (see **Fig. 8**). However, some overlap between malignant and benign groups was observed, which may be improved using 3D sonography.[17] Alcazar and colleagues[17] showed that, using 3D power Doppler sonography, vascular indices (VI, FI, and VFI) from suspicious adnexal areas such as thick papillary projections, solid areas, and mostly solid tumors were significantly higher in malignant tumors compared with benign tumors, which may reflect different angiogenic patterns.

Alcazar and Rodriquez[18] recommended that 3D sonography should be used in select patients in whom ovarian tumors are difficult to classify based on 2D parameters. In such cases, the 3D power Doppler technique may play a role in reducing the false-positive rate without substantially affecting the sensitivity. Using predetermined cutoffs for VI, FI, and VFI, their group was able to reduce the false-positive rate in this subset of adnexal masses by approximately one-third without substantially decreasing the sensitivity of the technique. The median VI (MVI), FI, and VFI were significantly higher among malignant tumors compared with nonmalignant lesions.[18] There were no differences in the RI, PI, and peak systolic velocity.[17,18]

An important contribution of color Doppler sonography using 3D volumetric sets is the ability to quantify the number of vessels and volume of flow within the area of interest. Qualitative and quantitative assessment of volume data is possible with color Doppler sonography. VOCAL offers a reliable, practical, noninvasive, and automatic method to calculate indices of vascularity, such as the VI, FI, and VFI.[2,19]

Other studies investigated quantitative vascular indices such as VI, FI, and VFI in a predetermined volume (1 mL) of benign and malignant tumors and found that malignancies had significantly higher values. One group found that the VI is less reliable than the FI because it is affected by the moment in the cardiac cycle in which the value was obtained.[20]

Using contrast enhancement and color Doppler sonography, Fleischer and colleagues[21] showed that both the baseline and absolute and maximum Doppler signals intensities (in decibels) were significantly higher in malignancies. However, the accuracy of CE-TVS in distinguishing benign from malignant ovarian masses was limited by its inability to distinguish borderline from benign lesion.[22,23]

Microbubble-enhanced sonography has the potential to provide a means to assess tumor response to various therapeutic measurements particularly in the light of the increased use of anti-angiogenic agents and the importance of monitoring tumor response, as has been described in hepatic tumors. Those responsive to chemotherapy show a marked reduction in vascularity preceding any decrease in volumetric dimensions.[7] In another study correlating the vascular indices derived from 3D TV color Doppler sonography with cervical tumor grade, a positive correlation of tumor size and grade with these parameters was reported.[24]

OVARIAN (ADNEXAL) TORSION

Ovarian (adnexal) torsion is a gynecologic emergency caused by twisting of the ovary on its pedicle, causing lymphatic and venous stasis, resulting in ovarian edema followed by ischemia and necrosis if left untreated.[25] Gray-scale sonography usually shows an enlarged ovary, small follicles around the periphery of the ovary, an ovarian solid/cystic mass, and free fluid in the cul-de-sac.[25–27] Color Doppler sonography may show a twisted ovarian pedicle present in torsed adnexae (**Fig. 9**).[28,29] Doppler sonography of the intraovarian vessels is helpful to predict ovarian viability with appropriate Doppler settings and adequate penetration of the ultrasound beam.[28–30] Completely absent arterial and venous ovarian blood flow are specific for torsion, although evidence of flow within the ovary does not exclude ovarian torsion. Several years ago, Fleischer and colleagues[29] reported that ovarian viability is marked by central venous blood flow within the ovary. A more recent retrospective review of 39 proven cases of torsed adnexae showed that approximately one-third had venous flow and more than half had arterial flow.[25]

Lee and colleagues[28] found that, in patients with surgically confirmed ovarian torsion, 88% had a twisted ovarian vascular pedicle detected on sonography. She suggested that flow within the vascular pedicle is a predictor of ovarian viability. Pena and colleagues[26] found that 60% of patients with surgically confirmed ovarian torsion had normal flow within the ovary on Doppler before surgery, concluding that Doppler is not a sensitive modality for diagnosing ovarian torsion and that normal flow does not rule out torsion. Auslender and colleagues[30] described coiling of the blood vessels where vessels are twisting and forming loops in the shape of a coil because of spiral rotation of the ovarian pedicle. They classified the groups of women based on flow within the ovary (arterial and venous, arterial only, and no flow) and suggested conservative versus surgical treatment based on these findings.[30]

It is postulated that microbubble-contrasted enhancement could provide information regarding ovarian perfusion and enhance visualization of the twisted pedicle seen in adnexal torsion. Thus, an area of relative ischemia might be detected before the onset of irreversible processes such as necrosis.

OVARIAN FUNCTION/FERTILITY DISORDERS

Approximately 20% to 30% of fertility disorders have been attributed to ovulatory disorders. Color Doppler sonography can provide information related to the physiology of folliculogenesis and overall ovarian flow. Flow parameters may correlate with ovarian function and endometrial development. Premature ovarian failure can be implied where there is reduced intraovarian flow, even though there may be a significant variation in flow during the ovulatory cycle.

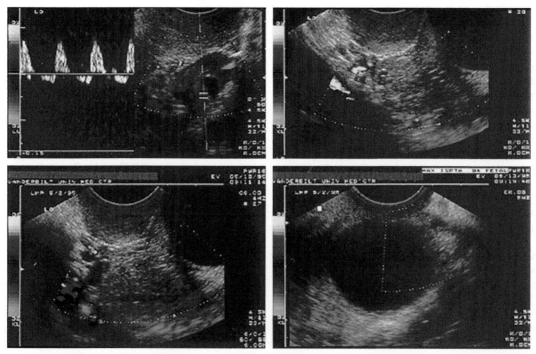

Fig. 9. TV color Doppler sonography of a torsed left ovary showing reversed diastolic flow (*top left*) in the twisted vascular pedicle (*top right* and *bottom left*). Paraovarian cyst (*bottom right*) was thought to precipitate ovarian torsion.

Color Doppler sonography helps to show intraovarian vascularity relative to follicular development, which can be used in optimization of the treatment of patients with ovulatory disorders (**Fig. 10**). Specifically, follicles that exhibit a ring of vascularity tend to produce fertilizable oocytes, whereas follicles that do not extrude an oocyte (luteinized unruptured follicles) are vascularized poorly.[31] 3D sonography also more accurately helps to determine follicle size in patients with infertility on ovulation induction medications.[32]

In infertility work-up, color Doppler sonography is used to assess endometrial development by depiction of its vascularity. An optimally primed endometrium usually contains several spiral vessels, whereas a poorly vascularized endometrium may preclude or delay attempts to perform embryo transfer. The relative receptivity of the endometrium can be quantitatively assessed using VOCAL 3D TV color Doppler sonography.[33]

Polycystic ovarian syndrome (PCOS) affects approximately 17% of women of reproductive age. In PCOS, the ovaries are morphologically characterized by having 10,12, or more follicles, measuring 2 to 9 mm, as well as increased ovarian volume, of 1 or both ovaries, measuring greater than or equal to 10 mL. However, in up to 20% to 30% of women with PCOS, the ovaries are of normal size. In these patients, 2D imaging may underestimate the number of follicles compared with 3D color Doppler sonography.[34] Lam and Raine-Fenning[34] concluded that 3D color Doppler sonography is an appropriate tool to assess and study the PCO because it provides a quantitative measurement of total ovarian and stromal echogenicity, volume, and blood flow in a way that is not possible with 2D TVS. In 2004, Wu and colleagues[35] described that, after certain treatments, there was a reduction in ovarian volume as well as a decrease in ovarian stromal blood flow during the early follicular phase in 40 clomiphene-resistant women with PCOS 3 months after laparoscopic ovarian drilling. Thus, the addition of color Doppler sonography to a morphologic finding could potentially improve understanding of the pathophysiology of this disorder and its response to various treatments.

UTERINE DISORDERS

Color Doppler sonography provides a means to assess several common uterine disorders such as fibroids, polyps, and vascular malformations.

Polyps

On gray-scale sonography, an endometrial polyp is shown as a round echogenic mass within the endometrium. A coronal view obtained by 3D sonography can more accurately identify polyps. Andreotti and colleagues[36] showed that a 3D reconstructed view of endometrium and adjacent myometrium was a valuable adjunct to conventional transvaginal sonography, providing additional information in up to half of patients who had abnormal findings on conventional 3D sonography.[37]

Color Doppler sonography is also useful in identifying blood flow to the polyp as a feeder vessel (see **Fig. 5**). La Torre and colleagues[38] showed that 3D sonography had high (88%) specificity for detecting endometrial polyps, and all polyps in their series were detected when 3D sonography was combined with saline infusion. Sylvester and colleagues[39] also showed increased specificity, with sensitivity and specificity of 97% and 11% for 2D imaging, 87% and 45% for 3D imaging, and 98% and 100% for 2D saline infusion sonography (SIS). In most patients, it is thought that the use of 3D color Doppler sonography may preclude the need for SIS. TV color Doppler sonography can be used to accurately distinguish endometrial polyps from submucosal fibroids by documentation of a single feeding vessel present in most polyps versus multiple peripherally arranged vessels in a submucosal fibroid (**Fig. 11**).[40]

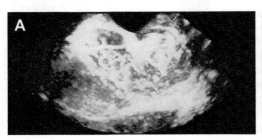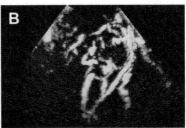

Fig. 10. 3D TV color Doppler sonography of a cervical fibroid immediately before (*A*) and after uterine artery embolization (UAE) (*B*). Significant flow remained after UAE, thought to be caused by the presence of ovarian collaterals.

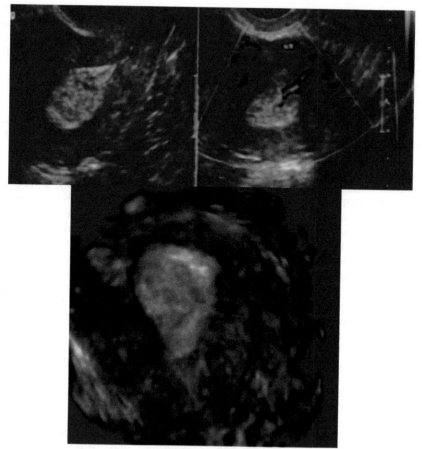

Fig. 11. TV gray-scale, power Doppler, and 3D coronal images showing a mass within the endometrial canal, which is slightly hypoechoic relative to the endometrium (the endometrium is echogenic in the secretory phase of the menstrual cycle) as well as the typical feeder vessel to the polyp.

Leiomyoma

Leiomyoma is the most common tumor of the uterus occurring in 20% to 25% of women older than 30 years. Location of fibroids within the uterus (submucosal, intramural, subserosal) is clinically important and, for this determination, 3D sonography is particularly useful. Color Doppler sonography and 3D imaging improve diagnostic accuracy to determine exact borders and relative vascularity.[41] In women with symptomatic uterine myomas who are considering uterine artery embolization (UAE), 3D sonography with Doppler may have an important role in evaluating the uterine vascularity before and after UAE by determining the vascularity of the fibroids and the presence of a pedunculated fibroid containing a vascular pedicle. Detection of ovarian collaterals to the fibroid by 3D color Doppler sonography is helpful before attempting UAE, because the presence of collateral vessels may negatively influence the outcome of embolization **(Fig. 12).**[42]

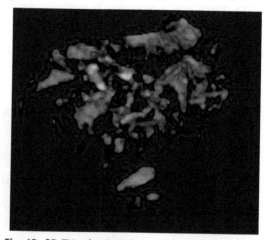

Fig. 12. 3D TV color Doppler sonography of the neo-vascularity within a malignant polyp, showing vessel irregularity and abnormal branching.

Vascular Abnormalities

3D color Doppler sonography is helpful in evaluating vascular abnormalities of the endometrium, myometrium, and parametrium. Uterine arteriovenous malformation (AVM) consists of vascular plexus of arteries and veins without an intervening capillary network. They are located in the myometrium and usually do not regress spontaneously with time. They may be congenital or acquired after uterine trauma, such as curettage, pelvic surgery, or previous treatment of gestational trophoblastic disease. Gray-scale morphology of uterine arteriovenous malformations is nonspecific. Color Doppler sonography is more consistent and specific and shows intense multidirectional turbulent flow/aliasing (**Fig. 13**).[43] Spectral analysis characteristically depicts a low-resistance, high-velocity arterial flow with low RI in the range of 0.25 to 0.55.[44] Peak systolic velocities recorded within the vascular malformation are also usually high, in the range of 40 to 100 cm/s.[45] However, Doppler findings associated with retained products of conception may be similar, with the most specific finding for AVM being the presence of arterialized venous flow.[46] Doppler sonography can also be used to monitor the response or recurrence of the vascular abnormality after embolization.

Uterine artery aneurysms or malformations are rare. A true aneurysm is usually congenital and may manifest as uterine bleeding from rupture during pregnancy in the puerperium. On gray scale, uterine artery aneurysm is a pulsating anechoic structure in the myometrium. Doppler sonography can diagnose an aneurysm with high sensitivity and specificity by depicting the dilatation of the uterine artery with characteristic arterial flow pattern. UAE is an effective treatment modality for uterine artery aneurysm and color Doppler sonography can be used for postembolization monitoring.

Uterine artery pseudoaneurysm (PSA) is an extraluminal collection of blood with turbulent flow that communicates with the parent vessel through a defect in the arterial wall. Uterine artery PSA is a rare vascular abnormality but is more common than aneurysm. It is usually a complication after pelvic surgery or trauma and can be diagnosed by arteriography or noninvasively by color Doppler sonography. Color Doppler imaging shows blood-filled cystic structures with varying colors caused by swirling movement of the arterial blood in different directions. Spectral analysis within the sac shows turbulent multidirectional arterial flow. In the neck of the PSA, the blood flow into the aneurysm in systole and out in diastole creates a characteristic bidirectional flow spectrum. Because of the small size of the uterine artery, it may be difficult to visualize the neck of the PSA, and, in such instances, arteriography is more useful.

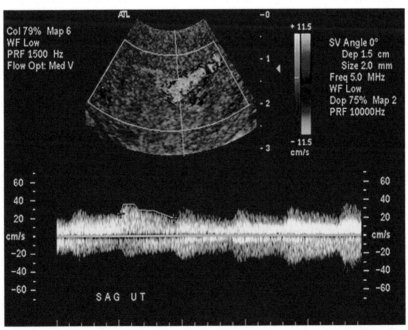

Fig. 13. TV color Doppler sonography arteriovenous malformation of a radial vessel associated with continuous vaginal bleeding in a patient after medical abortion. There is low-impedance, high-velocity flow within the abnormal vessels.

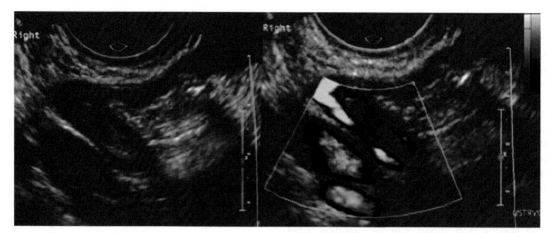

Fig. 14. Right ovarian vein thrombosis. Sagittal 2D gray-scale and power Doppler images of right adnexal region show an echogenic thrombus within the right ovarian vein and a small amount of flow around the thrombus on power Doppler images.

Distended paraovarian veins with sluggish or to-and-fro flow can be seen in women with nonspecific pelvic pain. This condition has been termed pelvic congestion syndrome. Occasionally, thrombi within a distended vessel are documented with TV color Doppler sonography (**Fig. 14**).

SUMMARY

2D and 3D color Doppler sonography afford depictions of ovarian and uterine vascularity that have many clinical applications, including improved detection and diagnosis of ovarian tumors, improved detection of ovarian (adnexal) torsion, uterine polyps, fibroids, and vascular malformations. When characterizing ovarian tumors, 3D sonography can evaluate vascular morphology of involved vessels and quantitate the relative vascularity of the area of interest. There may also be potential value in the use of contrast-enhanced sonography to detect early ovarian carcinoma and monitor response to treatment.

REFERENCES

1. Fleischer AC, Milam MR, Crispens MA, et al. Sonographic depiction of intratumoral vascularity with 2- and 3-dimensional color Doppler techniques. J Ultrasound Med 2005;24:533–7.
2. Raine-Fenning NJ, Campbell BK, Clewes JS, et al. The reliability of virtual organ computer-aided analysis (VOCAL) for the semiquantification of ovarian, endometrial and subendometrial perfusion. Ultrasound Obstet Gynecol 2003;22:633–9.
3. Fleischer AC, Lyshchik A, Jones HW, et al. Contrast-enhanced transvaginal sonography of benign versus malignant ovarian masses: preliminary findings. J Ultrasound Med 2008;27: 1011–21.
4. Fleischer AC, Lyshchik A, Andreotti RF. Advances in sonographic detection of ovarian cancer: depiction of tumor neovascularity with microbubbles. AJR Am J Roentgenol 2010;194:343–8.
5. Marret H, Sauget S, Giraudeau B, et al. Contrast-enhanced sonography helps in discrimination of benign from malignant adnexal masses. J Ultrasound Med 2004;23:1629–42.
6. Testa AC, Ferrandina G, Fruscella E, et al. The use of contrasted transvaginal sonography in the diagnosis of gynecologic diseases: a preliminary study. J Ultrasound Med 2005;24:1267–78.
7. Hwang M, Neirmann K, Lyshchik A, et al. Sonographic assessment of tumor response from in vivo models to clinical applications. Ultrasound Q 2009; 25:175–83.
8. Cohen LS, Escobar PF, Scharm C, et al. Three-dimensional power Doppler ultrasound improves the diagnostic accuracy for ovarian cancer prediction. Gynecol Oncol 2001;82(1):40–8.
9. Raine-Fenning NJ, Campbell BK, Clewes JS, et al. The interobserver reliability of three-dimensional power Doppler data acquisition within the female pelvis. Ultrasound Obstet Gynecol 2004;23:501–8.
10. Kurjac A, Shalan H, Kupesic S, et al. Transvaginal color Doppler sonography in assessment of pelvic tumor vascularity. Ultrasound Obstet Gynecol 1993;3:137–54.
11. Fleischer AC, Rogers WH, Rao BK, et al. Assessment of ovarian tumor vascularity with transvaginal color Doppler sonography. J Ultrasound Med 1991;10:563–8.
12. Kurjak A, Kupesic S, Sparac V, et al. Three-dimensional ultrasonographic and power Doppler

characterization of ovarian lesions. Ultrasound Obstet Gynecol 2000;16:365–71.

13. Geomini PM, Kluivers KB, Moret E, et al. Evaluation of adnexal masses with three-dimensional ultrasonography. Obstet Gynecol 2006;108:1167–75.

14. Guerriero S, Ajossa S, Piras S, et al. Three dimensional quantification of tumor vascularity as a tertiary test after B-mode and power Doppler evaluation for detection of ovarian cancer. J Ultrasound Med 2007;26:1271–8.

15. Timmerman D, Testa AC, Bourne T, et al. Simple ultrasound-based rules for the diagnosis of ovarian cancer. Ultrasound Obstet Gynecol 2008;31:681–90.

16. Wilson WD, Valet AS, Andreotti RF, et al. Sonographic quantification of ovarian tumor vascularity. J Ultrasound Med 2006;25(12):1577–81.

17. Alcazar JL, Merce LT, Manero MG. Three dimensional power Doppler vascular sampling. A new method for predicting ovarian cancer in vascularized complex adnexal masses. J Ultrasound Med 2005;24:689–96.

18. Alcazar JL, Rodriguez D. Three-dimensional power Doppler vascular sonographic sampling for predicting ovarian cancer in cystic-solid and solid vascularized masses. J Ultrasound Med 2009;28:275–81.

19. Pairleitner H, Steiner H, Hasenoehrl G, et al. Three dimensional power Doppler sonography: imaging and quantifying blood flow and vascularization. Ultrasound Obstet Gynecol 1999;14:139–43.

20. Kudla MJ, Alcazar JL. Spatiotemporal image correlation using high-definition flow. A new method for assessing ovarian vascularization. J Ultrasound Med 2010;29:1469–74.

21. Fleischer AC, Lyshchik A, Jones H, et al. Contrast enhanced transvaginal sonography of benign versus malignant ovarian masses. J Ultrasound Med 2008;27:1011–8.

22. Testa AC, Timmerman D, Van Belle V, et al. Intravenous contrast ultrasound examination using contrast-tuned imaging (CnTI™) and the contrast medium SonoVue® for discrimination between benign and malignant adnexal masses with solid components. Ultrasound Obstet Gynecol 2009;34:699–710.

23. Veyer L, Marret H, Bleuzen A, et al. Preoperative diagnosis of ovarian tumors using pelvic contrast-enhanced sonography. J Ultrasound Med 2010; 29(7):1041–9.

24. Testa AC, Gerrandina G, Distefano M, et al. Color Doppler velocimetry and three-dimensional color power angiography of cervical carcinoma. Ultrasound Obstet Gynecol 2004;24:441–52.

25. Shadinger LL, Andreotti RF, Kurian RL. Preoperative sonographic and clinical characteristics as predictors of ovarian torsion. J Ultrasound Med 2008;27: 4278–97.

26. Pena JE, Ufberg D, Cooney N, et al. Usefulness of Doppler sonography in the diagnosis of ovarian torsion. Fertil Steril 2000;73:1047–50.

27. Smorgick N, Maymon R, Mendelovic S, et al. Torsion of normal adnexa in postmenarcheal women: can ultrasound indicate an ischemic process? Ultrasound Obstet Gynecol 2008;31:338–41.

28. Lee EJ, Kwon HC, Joo HJ, et al. Diagnosis of ovarian torsion with color Doppler sonography: depiction of twisted vascular pedicle. J Ultrasound Med 1998; 17:83–9.

29. Fleischer AC, Stein S, Cullinan J, et al. Color Doppler sonography of adnexal torsion. J Ultrasound Med 1995;14:523–8.

30. Auslender R, Shen O, Kaufman Y, et al. Doppler and gray scale sonographic classification of adnexal torsion. Ultrasound Obstet Gynecol 2009;34:208–11.

31. Merce LT, Garves D, Barco MJ, et al. Intraovarian Doppler velocimetry in ovulatory, dysovulatory and anovulatory cycles. Ultrasound Obstet Gynecol 1992;2(3):197–202.

32. Kupesic S, Kurjak A. Predictors of IVF outcome by three-dimensional ultrasound. Hum Reprod 2002; 17:950–5.

33. Raine-Fenning N, Fleischer AC. Clarifying the role of three-dimensional transvaginal sonography in reproductive medicine: an evidence-based appraisal. J Exp Clin Assist Reprod 2005;2:10.

34. Lam P, Raine-Fenning N. The role of three-dimensional ultrasonography in polycystic ovary syndrome. Hum Reprod 2006;21(9):2209–15.

35. Wu MH, Huang MF, Tsai SJ, et al. Effects of laparoscopic ovarian drilling on young adult women with polycystic ovarian syndrome. J Am Assoc Gynecol Laparosc 2004;11:184–90.

36. Andreotti RF, Fleischer AC, Mason LE. 3-Dimensional sonography of endometrium and adjacent myometrium preliminary observations. J Ultrasound Med 2006;25:1313–9.

37. Benacerraf BR, Shipp TD, Bromley B. Which patients benefit from a 3D reconstructed coronal view of the uterus added to standard routine 2D pelvic sonography? AJR Am J Roentgenol 2008;190:626–9.

38. La Torre R, De Felipe C, De Angelis C, et al. Transvaginal sonographic evaluation of endometrial polyps: a comparison with 2-dimensional and 3-dimensional contrast sonography. Clin Exp Obstet Gynecol 1999;26:171–3.

39. Sylvester C, Child TJ, Tulandi T, et al. Prospective study to evaluate the efficacy of 2- and 3-D sonohysterography in women with intrauterine lesions. Fertil Steril 2003;79:1222–5.

40. Fleischer AC, Shappell HW. Color Doppler sonohysterography of endometrial polyps and submucosal fibroids. J Ultrasound Med 2003;22:601–4.

41. Bragg AC, Angtuaco TL. Three-dimensional gynecologic ultrasound. Ultrasound Clin 2010;5:299–311.

42. Fleischer AC, Donnelly EF, Campbell MG. 3-Dimensional color Doppler sonography before and after fibroid embolization. J Ultrasound Med 2000;19:701–5.

43. Pope S, Fleischer AC, Bream PR. Intramyometrial AVM. J Wom Imag 2003;5:79–82.
44. Secil M, Dogra V. Color flow Doppler evaluation of uterus and ovaries and its optimization techniques. Ultrasound Clin 2008;3(3):461–82.
45. Timmerman D, Wauters DJ, Van Calenbergh S. Color Doppler imaging is a valuable tool for the diagnosis and management of uterine vascular malformations. Ultrasound Obstet Gynecol 2003; 21:570–7.
46. Jain K, Fogata M. Retained products of conception mimicking a large endometrial AVM: complete resolution following spontaneous abortion. J Clin Ultrasound 2007;35:42–7.

Pediatric Gynecologic Ultrasound

Brian D. Coley, MD

KEYWORDS

- Ultrasound • Children • Congenital anomalies • Masses
- Puberty

As in adults, ultrasound is the first and often most definitive imaging modality for the evaluation of the female pelvis. Common reasons for clinical referral include evaluation of pelvic pain or a pelvic mass, abnormalities of puberty, and disorders of sexual development. An understanding of the basics of gynecologic embryology is necessary to understand congenital malformations that often predispose to these clinical scenarios.

TECHNIQUE

Transabdominal imaging is the mainstay of pediatric pelvic imaging and is adequate for most clinical indications. As with any other study, the transducer frequency used depends on patient size. Infants and small children can be imaged with high-frequency curvilinear or linear transducers, whereas older or larger patients may require low-frequency sector transducers for adequate visualization of pelvic structures. A full bladder allows an acoustic window into the pelvis and displaces bowel out of the pelvis.[1] When oral fluids are inadequate or too slow, intravenous fluid administration or bladder catheterization and filling can achieve bladder filling.

Transvaginal imaging is often not considered in pediatric patients but can be valuable in solving problems in the older adolescent and young adult. Patients who are nonvirginal or who use tampons and who consent or assent to the procedure are candidates. Most adolescents tolerate transvaginal scanning and are often appreciative of being able to forgo the discomfort of bladder filling. Although transvaginal scanning can provide superior imaging of the uterus and ovaries, transabdominal imaging should still be performed (even if the bladder is not optimally distended) to give a broader view of the pelvis and cul-de-sac.

Transperineal imaging is valuable in evaluating the external genitalia, labia, and introitus.[1] High-frequency linear or curvilinear transducers can provide valuable images and should be covered as with transvaginal imaging. Although not widely used in most pediatric practices, three-dimensional imaging with multiplanar reconstructions can be beneficial in the evaluation of uterine anomalies and may obviate the need for MR imaging.[2,3]

When evaluating a patient for structural anomalies, questions of sexual differentiation, or menstrual disorders, it is essential to evaluate the adrenal glands and urinary system. Associated anomalies are common and can provide important additional information to the treating clinician.

NORMAL ANATOMY
Newborn and Infant

The newborn ovary can sometimes be difficult to visualize but, with patience and persistence, they are visible in most cases. Newborn ovaries may measure up to 3.6 mL in volume and commonly have follicles measuring up to 9 mm.[1] The newborn uterus has a volume up to 4 mL with a characteristic "spade" shape due to a prominent cervix[1]; a visible endometrium is common (**Fig. 1**). As maternal hormones wane, the ovaries and uterus take on their infantile appearance that will persist until the prepubertal period (**Fig. 2**). Ovarian volumes in the infant should be less than 2 mL; follicles are still seen in up to half of patients and should be considered normal.[1,4] The uterus similarly decreases in size and attains a tubular

The author has nothing to disclose.
Department of Radiology, Cincinnati Children's Hospital Medical Center, 3333 Burnet Avenue, MLC-5031, Cincinnati, OH 45229, USA
E-mail address: brian.coley@cchmc.org

Ultrasound Clin 7 (2012) 107–121
doi:10.1016/j.cult.2011.10.001

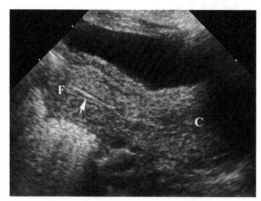

Fig. 1. Normal newborn uterus. Longitudinal sonogram of the pelvis shows a uterus with a cervix (C) that is more prominent than the fundus (F). Visible endometrial stripe from maternal hormonal stimulation (*arrow*).

shape with similar cervical and fundal diameters.[5] Decreased hormone levels also lead to a disappearance of a visible endometrial stripe.

Puberty

In the few years before the onset of puberty, both the ovaries and uterus gradually enlarge. In the years before menarche, ovarian volumes range between 2 and 4 mL. By the onset of menarche, the ovaries become more ovoid with volumes greater than 4 mL with multiple follicles.[1,4] With approaching menarche, the uterine fundus begins to enlarge and attain the mature "pear" shape (**Fig. 3**). Once menses begin and hormonal stimulation increases, the endometrium proliferates, becomes more sonographically conspicuous, and undergoes cyclical changes.[1]

CONGENITAL ANOMALIES

Abnormalities of genital development come to clinical attention in the newborn period when there are questions about ambiguous genitalia or in the pubertal period when there are abnormalities of menstruation. The detailed embryology of the genital tract is not the purpose of this article, but a basic understanding is necessary for the understanding and interpretation of imaging findings.

In the absence of a Y chromosome and in the presence of two X chromosomes, the embryonic and fetal gonad differentiates into an ovary. A missing X chromosome may lead to streak ovaries as are often found in Turner syndrome.[1]

The uterus, cervix, upper two-thirds of the vagina, and the fallopian tubes arise from the müllerian duct system (MDS). The paired müllerian or paramesonephric ducts normally undergo longitudinal fusion to form a single upper vagina and uterus. The distal vagina is formed from the genital ridge. Fusion with the upper vagina and degeneration of the intervening transverse tissue results in a normal vagina and introitus. Congenital anomalies can thus be thought of in terms of failure of longitudinal or transverse anomalies of fusion, separation, and regression.[6,7] Additional important features include whether there is obstruction and concomitant ovarian, renal, and skeletal anomalies.

Uterus

The prevalence of MDS malformations is unclear, but it is approximately 0.4% in unselected patients. It is higher among women with infertility and a history of recurrent miscarriage.[7,8] MDS anomalies are generally classified according to the American Society of Reproductive Medicine (**Fig. 4**).[9] Although useful, this classification sometimes fails to allow adequate description of multiple anomalies of the genital system, making accurate description of imaging findings essential to properly guide clinical care.

Complete aplasia of the uterus and upper vagina is referred to as the Mayer-Rokitansky-Küster-Hauser syndrome (MRKH) and represents up to

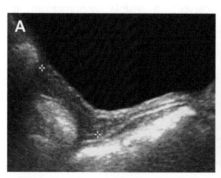
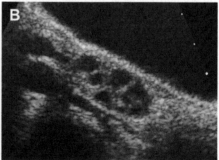

Fig. 2. Normal prepubertal uterus and ovaries. (*A*) Longitudinal sonogram of the pelvis in a 5-year-old girl shows a normal uterus (*cursors*) with the fundus and cervix of similar diameters. There is no visible endometrium. (*B*) The ovary in the same patient has multiple small follicles, which are normal.

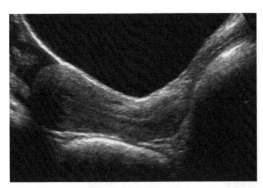

Fig. 3. Normal pubertal uterus. Longitudinal sonogram in a 14-year-old girl shows a normal uterus with a fundal diameter greater than the cervix. A thin endometrial stripe is visible.

10% of MDS malformations.[7] These young women have normal secondary sexual characteristics and present with primary amenorrhea.[10] MRKH is usually an isolated malformation without any specific inheritance pattern.[6,11] When associated with renal, ear, and skeletal abnormalities, this is referred to as müllerian duct aplasia, unilateral renal aplasia, cervicothoracic somite dysplasia (MURCS) or MRKH type II.[11–13] Ultrasound fails to demonstrate a uterus, but the ovaries are typically normal (**Fig. 5**). Evaluation of the urinary system may disclose unilateral agenesis or other abnormalities.

Failure of one of the müllerian ducts to develop results in a unicornuate uterus. A rudimentary horn is usually present, may or may not contain functional endometrium, and may or may not communicate with the normal uterine horn.[14,15] If there is functional endometrial tissue and the rudimentary horn is obstructed, menstrual products will accumulate and patients may present with pain, mass, or endometriosis symptoms. Associated ipsilateral renal anomalies are seen in as many as 50% of patients, and range from simple collecting system duplication to aplasia.[6] At ultrasound, the normal horn may appear normal, elongated, or laterally displaced (**Fig. 6**). The ultrasound appearance of the rudimentary horn depends on the degree of maldevelopment and presence of obstruction.

If there is failure of resorption of the dividing septum or incomplete fusion of the two müllerian ducts, the result is varying degrees of uterine and vaginal duplication. Uterus didelphys results from complete nonfusion, leading to two separate uteri, cervices, and vaginas without any communication (**Fig. 7**). Lesser degrees of fusion lead to varying degrees of bicornuate uterus, with one or two cervices and a single vagina (**Fig. 8**). Failure of

resorption of the longitudinal uterovaginal septum leads to a septated uterus.[7,13] An arcuate uterus represents the mildest manifestation of this sequence and it is debatable whether this should just be considered a normal variant because there is no real clinical implication.

Differentiation of uterine fusion anomalies (bicornuate) from resorption anomalies (septate) relies on evaluation of the contour of the uterine fundus. A smooth, normally convex outer myometrium indicates proper uterine fusion and, thus, tissue separating the uterine cavities a residual septum. With bicornuate uteri, there is a cleft between the two uterine horns creating a concave fundal contour.[16] Coronal imaging is best able to show this contour, and MR imaging has traditionally been touted as being superior to ultrasound for this evaluation. Recent work suggests that three-dimension ultrasound is as reliable as MR imaging in defining uterine anomalies because it allows image reconstruction in the coronal plane and improved visualization of the uterine cavity (or cavities) and the contour of the fundus.[2]

Vagina

As previously discussed, atresia of the upper vagina accompanies MRKH. Hypoplasia or aplasia may also rarely occur with Turner syndrome.[13] Other MDS anomalies are concomitant vaginal obstruction from residual longitudinal or transverse vaginal septa. Congenital abnormalities of the urogenital, sinus-producing, distal vaginal atresia that present in the newborn are less common; however, they are seen in patients with a stenotic or obstructed urogenital sinus or cloacal malformation.[17,18] The transverse vaginal septum between the upper and lower vagina normally resorbs leading to a single vaginal cavity; persistence of this septum leads to vaginal obstruction. An imperforate hymen is a more common cause of vaginal obstruction, and may present in neonates or pubertal patients.[16,19,20] Patients present with a pelvic mass from distension of the vagina with fluid (hydrocolpos) or blood (hematocolpos); the uterus may also be filled (hydrometrocolpos or hematometrocolpos). The fallopian tubes may also be dilated from retrograde filling. With more severe distension, there may be bladder outlet obstruction or ureteral obstruction and hydronephrosis.

Ultrasound shows echogenic fluid in the vagina outlining the cervix (**Fig. 9**). Depending on the pressure in the vagina and cervical competence, there may also be dilatation of the uterus. Occasionally, it may be difficult to differentiate the distended vagina from the uterus. Transperineal

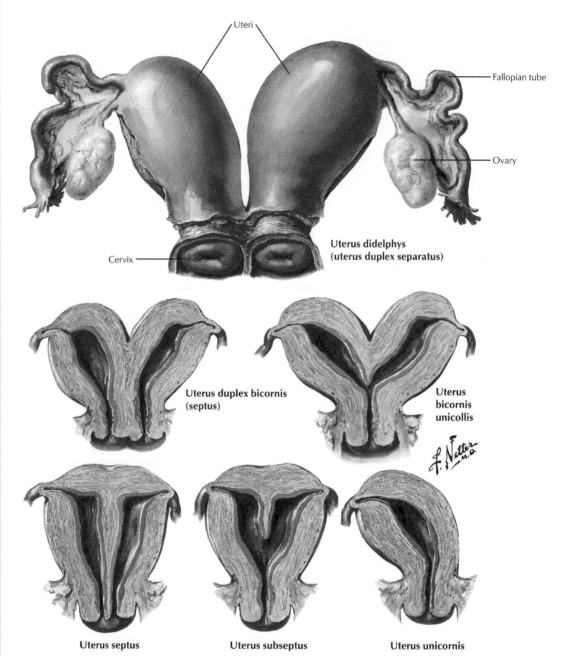

Fig. 4. Congenital uterine anomalies. (Netter illustration from www.netterimages.com. © Elsevier, Inc. All rights reserved.)

scanning helps to delineate the thickness of the obstructing membrane, which helps distinguish a transverse septum from an imperforate hymen (Fig. 10), although physical examination is often sufficient for this. Additionally, with a transverse septum, the inferior margin of the dilated vagina may be superior to the inferior margin of the full urinary bladder; whereas, with imperforate hymen, the dilated vagina extends more inferiorly.[13]

DISORDERS OF SEXUAL DEVELOPMENT

A disorder of sexual development (DSD) exists when a child's phenotype cannot be definitely determined or when chromosomal gender does not match with phenotypic gender.[21,22] This occurs in approximately 1 in 6000 births[22] and can be divided into four main categories[16,21,23]: gonadal dysgenesis, true hermaphroditism (presence of ovotestis), male pseudohermaphroditism

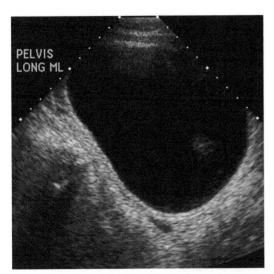

Fig. 5. Mayer-Rokitansky-Küster-Hauser syndrome. Longitudinal sonogram of the pelvis in a 15-year-old girl with secondary amenorrhea shows no identifiable uterus. The ovaries and kidneys were normal.

(46,XY; two testes), and female pseudohermaphroditism (46,XX; two ovaries). Ultrasound plays a central role in diagnosis by determining whether the uterus is present and by evaluating the appearance of the gonads.[23] Genitography can help in the evaluation of the urethra and whether any fistulas coexist. Early evaluation of DSD is important for sex determination and these conditions can have significant psychosocial impact for both parents and patients.

Patients with pure gonadal dysgenesis are phenotypic females and present for evaluation due to primary amenorrhea. An underdeveloped uterus will be present but no normal gonads will be seen. Patients with mixed gonadal dysgenesis have a mosaic 45,XO/46,XY karyotype and ambiguous genitalia; one gonad is a testis and one is a streak ovary.[16,21] A uterus is usually present, although it may be unicornuate opposite the side of the testis (**Fig. 11**).[21] Patients with gonadal dysgenesis are at an increased risk for developing neoplasia, particularly gonadoblastoma.[23] Karyotypic males with gonadal dysgenesis are also at an increased risk for Wilms tumor and should undergo ultrasound surveillance.[23]

True hermaphroditism represents less than 10% of DSD.[16] Karyotypes are most commonly 46,XX, but others have a mosaic 46,XY pattern.[21] External genitalia are ambiguous. Ultrasound will demonstrate a uterus. The gonads can be an ovary and a testis, an ovotestis on one side and an ovary or testis on the other, or bilateral ovotestes. The presence of small cysts within a heterogeneous, otherwise solid, gonad indicates follicles within an ovotestis.

Male pseudohermaphrodites have a normal male karyotype with varying degrees of feminized external genitalia (bifid scrotum, small phallus, hypospadias). The testes are present, but may be undescended or located in unfused labioscrotal folds. The underlying cause is a failure of androgen production or end-organ androgen insensitivity, which can be complete or partial. Patients with complete androgen insensitivity are phenotypically female, and may not present until there is concern for primary amenorrhea.[21] Müllerian structures are absent at sonography so there will be no uterus. Normal testes are usually

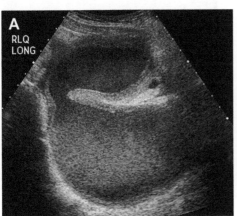

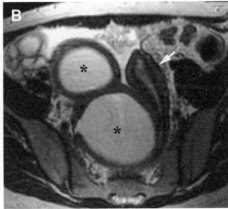

Fig. 6. Obstructed uterine horn. (*A*) Transabdominal sonogram in a 14-year-old girl with cyclic abdominal pain and a palpable mass shows a large lobular right pelvic mass with echogenic debris. No right kidney was found. A normal uterine horn was not convincingly seen. (*B*) Axial T2-weighted MR image shows the obstructed right uterine horn (*asterisks*) and a normal-appearing left uterine horn (*arrow*). MR imaging confirmed right renal agenesis.

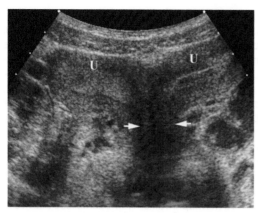

Fig. 7. Uterus didelphys. Transverse sonogram in a 7-year-old girl shows two separate uteri (U) and two separate cervices (*arrows*). The vaginas were also completely separate.

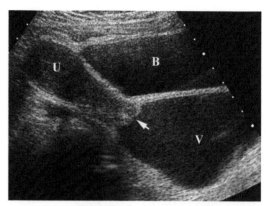

Fig. 9. Imperforate hymen and hydrocolpos. Longitudinal sonogram in a patient with cyclical pain but no menses shows debris-filled fluid distending the vagina (V) that outlines the cervix (*arrow*). The uterus (U) is normal. B, bladder.

demonstrable, but may be malpositioned. Given the risk of neoplasia in these undescended testes, they are often removed.

Female pseudohermaphrodites have a normal female karyotype with varying degrees of virilized external genitalia (labioscrotal fusion, clitiromegaly). The most common cause is congenital adrenal hyperplasia (CAH) with an associated 21-hydroxylase deficiency.[23–25] Ultrasound shows a normal uterus and ovaries. The adrenal glands are abnormally thick and long with a lobulated or cerebriform surface that is characteristic of CAH **(Fig. 12).**[26]

DISORDERS OF MENSES AND MATURATION
Precocious Puberty

Despite the trend for earlier development of secondary sexual characteristics and the onset of menses,[27] precocious puberty is still defined

when this occurs before 8 years of age.[28,29] True isosexual (or central) precocious puberty is due to premature elevation of gonadotropin levels resulting in the development of secondary sexual characteristics and menses.[30] This activation of the hypothalamic-pituitary-gonadal axis is most often idiopathic but can be secondary to structural abnormalities of the central nervous system and tumors (most commonly a hypothalamic hamartoma).[30] Peripheral precocious puberty is less common and results from peripheral production of estrogens resulting in ovarian follicular development and uterine growth, along with

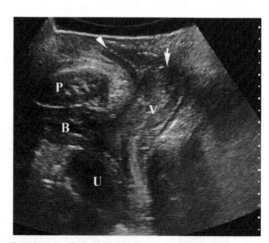

Fig. 10. Distal vaginal atresia. Transperineal sonogram in an 8-year-old girl without an external vaginal opening on physical examination. The distal end (*arrow*) of the vagina (V) could be clearly delineated posterior to the urethra (*arrowhead*). Ultrasound guided the location of the surgical incision made for repair. B, bladder; P, pubis symphysis U, uterus.

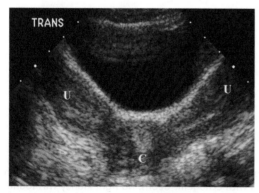

Fig. 8. Bicornuate uterus. Transverse sonogram in a 12-year-old girl shows two separate uteri (U) leading to a single cervix (C).

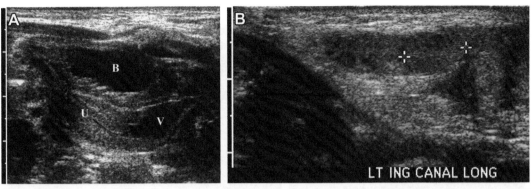

Fig. 11. Mixed gonadal dysgenesis. (*A*) Longitudinal sonogram in a newborn with ambiguous external genitalia shows a normal uterus (U) posterior to the bladder (B). There is a small amount of fluid in the vagina (V). (*B*) Sonogram of the left inguinal region shows a gonad (*cursors*) that looks more like a testis than an ovary, which was confirmed at surgery.

secondary sexual characteristics. However, gonadotropin levels are normal so ovulation and true menstruation does not occur.

Central causes are best evaluated by MR imaging, whereas causes of peripheral precocious puberty are best evaluated by ultrasound. Peripheral causes include functioning ovarian cysts, ovarian neoplasms (granulosa cell tumors, thecomas), CAH and adrenal neoplasms, and the McCune-Albright syndrome. Ultrasound also allows evaluation of the effects of hormonal stimulation by determining if there is ovarian enlargement and follicular stimulation, and uterine fundal development and endometrial proliferation (**Fig. 13**). Ultrasound can also confirm the effect of treatment with the return of the uterus and ovaries to a normal prepubertal appearance.[30,31]

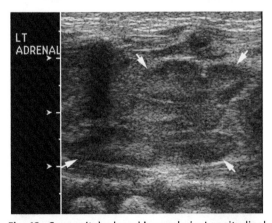

Fig. 12. Congenital adrenal hyperplasia. Longitudinal sonogram of the left-upper quadrant in a newborn with virilized external genitalia shows an enlarged adrenal gland (*arrows*) with multiple folds characteristic of this condition. The right adrenal gland looked the same.

Isolated vaginal bleeding in the absence of the development of secondary sexual characteristics (isolated precocious menarche) is uncommon and it should raise suspicion for neoplasia (see later discussion), vaginal foreign body, and sexual abuse. Vaginal foreign bodies usually appear echogenic at ultrasound, although appearances vary depending on the object.[6,13]

Amenorrhea

Primary amenorrhea indicates failure of menstruation by the age of 16 years. Secondary amenorrhea indicates that menses had begun but have subsequently ceased. The most common causes of primary amenorrhea are gonadal dysgenesis, MRKH syndrome, failure of the hypothalamic-pituitary axis, virilizing adrenal neoplasm, polycystic ovarian syndrome (PCOS), and gonadal failure from prior chemotherapy.[32] As discussed previously, failure to start menses may be the first indication of a DSD in a phenotypically normal girl.

Secondary amenorrhea may result from central nervous system tumors interrupting normal gonadotropin cycles, virilizing ovarian or adrenal tumors, and PCOS. Young women with markedly reduced body fat from athletics or dance, or from anorexia, may also experience secondary amenorrhea.[26]

Ultrasound appearances in primary and secondary amenorrhea depend on the underlying cause. The presence or absence of the uterus and ovaries can be evaluated and an assessment of hormonal stimulation can be made (**Fig. 14**). The ovaries in patients with PCOS are classically described as enlarged (>10 mL), with more than 12 follicles in each ovary, and abnormally echogenic stroma (**Fig. 15**).[33]

A

B

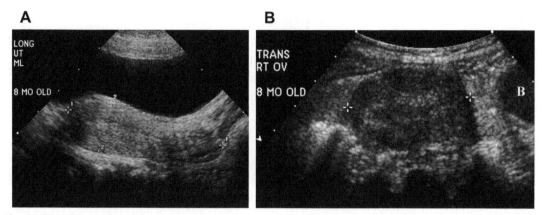

Fig. 13. Precocious puberty due to granulosa cell tumor. (*A*) Longitudinal sonogram in an 8-month-old girl with precocious puberty shows an enlarged uterus (*cursors*) with fundal development and a visible endometrium indicating hormonal stimulation. (*B*) Transverse sonogram shows a solid mass enlarging the right ovary (*cursors*). After resection, the patient's pubertal status returned to normal and the uterus took on the expected prepubertal tubular shape.

PELVIC MASS
Vagina and Uterus

Rhabdomyosarcoma is the most common pediatric genitourinary tract neoplasm, with one incidence peak in young childhood and one in adolescence.[16] In girls, the most common site of origin is the upper vagina. Patients usually present with vaginal bleeding, but there may also be a palpable or visible mass. Direct invasion to the uterus may cause uterine obstruction and local pelvic spread may produce ureteral obstruction and hydronephrosis.[13,26] Less common neoplasms include endodermal sinus tumors, adenocarcinoma, and leiomyosarcoma. Ultrasound of these masses is nonspecific, showing a soft tissue mass with or without cystic areas of necrosis (**Fig. 16**). Local invasion may be demonstrable, although, in some cases, this may be better evaluated with MR imaging.

Primary uterine tumors are uncommon in the pediatric age group. Leiomyomas are typically hypoechoic and are well circumscribed. Diffuse or focal involvement with non-Hodgkin lymphoma is a rare cause of uterine enlargement.[34]

Ovaries

Cysts
Follicular cysts are the most common benign ovarian mass.[35,36] In the neonate, these cysts

Fig. 14. Amenorrhea from hypothalamic-pituitary axis failure. Longitudinal sonogram of a 16-year-old girl with primary amenorrhea shows a small prepubertal uterus with no fundal development or visible endometrium. The ovaries were present but also appeared infantile.

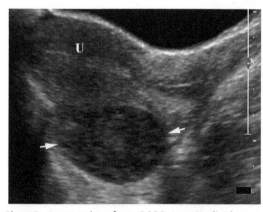

Fig. 15. Amenorrhea from PCOS. Longitudinal sonogram of the pelvis in an overweight teenager with facial hair shows an enlarged ovary (*arrows*) posterior to the uterus (U) with innumerable small follicles and echogenic central stroma.

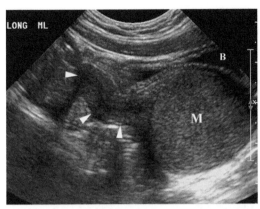

Fig. 16. Vaginal rhabdomyosarcoma. Longitudinal sonogram of the pelvis in an infant with vaginal bleeding and a visible mass shows a large, solid mass (M) within the vagina displacing the bladder (B) anteriorly. There was internal vascularity with color Doppler. The uterus (*arrowheads*) appears normal.

arise because of maternal hormonal stimulation and may be seen prenatally. Sonographically, these appear as simple cysts, often with small peripheral daughter cysts that confirm their follicular origin. Most cysts less than 4 cm will spontaneously resolve over several months.[37] Larger cysts may hemorrhage (**Fig. 17**) and cysts greater than 4 cm are thought to be at increased risk of ovarian torsion (see later discussion).[37,38] In postpubertal girls, normal dominant maturing follicles may measure up to 3 cm. Anovulatory functional cysts may measure up to 5 cm in diameter. In a recent consensus panel report,[39] simple-appearing cysts in reproductive age women up to 5 cm were thought not to warrant any specific follow-up given the very low malignant potential.

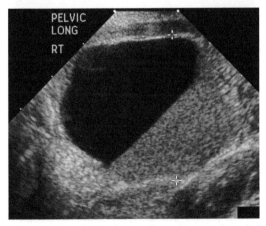

Fig. 17. Hemorrhagic neonatal ovarian cyst. Longitudinal sonogram of the right pelvis shows a large cyst (*cursors*) with a fluid-debris level indicating a hemorrhagic ovarian cyst. A separate right ovary was not found and the left ovary was normal.

Cysts between 5 cm and 7 cm should be followed, and those over 7 cm should be further evaluated with MR imaging or surgery.

Hemorrhagic cysts can create varying imaging appearances depending on the time since the hemorrhage has occurred. Early on, internal hemorrhage may give the cyst a solid appearance, although color Doppler will show no internal vascularity. With time, a debris fluid level, or a lacelike pattern of internal fibrinous strands may develop (**Fig. 18**)[40] with the complex mass decreasing in size over time and eventually disappearing.

Paraovarian cysts appear the same as other simple cysts; they arise within the broad ligament and they may be seen in adolescents. Peritoneal inclusion cysts form in women with adhesions from prior surgery or pelvic inflammatory disease that cause ovarian fluid to become loculated and trapped, instead of becoming resorbed by the peritoneal cavity.[41] Ultrasound shows a cystic mass that may be septated, but the findings are not specific.

An unusual cause of bilateral ovarian cysts is associated with hypothyroidism and precocious puberty, termed Van Wyk-Grumbach syndrome.[42] It is thought that elevated levels of thyroid-stimulating hormone may cause stimulation of follicle, stimulating hormone receptors leading to ovarian stimulation. These cysts may appear complex and can mimic a solid neoplasm, so appreciation of the imaging findings with the proper clinical context is essential to avoid unnecessary intervention. Appropriate thyroid hormone replacement leads to resolution of the cysts and associated symptoms.

Endometriosis is usually diagnosed in young adulthood but can affect younger women and adolescents,[43] especially those with uterine obstruction malformations. Ultrasound is often normal. Endometriomas have a similar appearance to that of older patients, appearing as a complex ovarian or paraovarian mass with low-level internal echoes.[44]

Cystic neoplasms

Cystic teratomas are the most common benign pediatric ovarian neoplasm.[45] More than 90% are benign and, thus, cured with surgical resection. Tumors are generally unilateral, but contralateral masses may be present in up to 20%. Many are discovered incidentally or present with an asymptomatic mass. Larger lesions may lead to ovarian torsion or undergo hemorrhage leading to pain. An unusual presentation of ovarian teratomas is encephalitis caused by anti–N-methyl-d-aspartate (NMDA) receptor antibodies. Neural

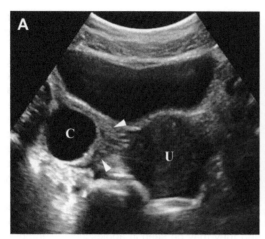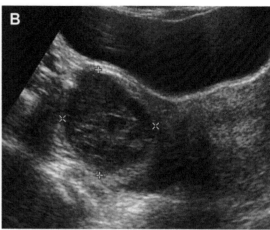

Fig. 18. Ovarian cyst with interval hemorrhage. (*A*) Transverse sonogram of a teenage girl with right pelvic pain shows a cyst versus dominant follicle (C) surrounded by normal ovarian tissue (*arrowheads*). U, uterus. (*B*) Two days later she had increasing pain and ultrasound showed enlargement of the previous simple cyst (*cursors*) with internal complexity. Laparoscopy confirmed a hemorrhagic cyst without torsion.

tissue present in some teratomas induce cross-reacting antibodies that attack NMDA receptors in the hippocampus causing limbic encephalitis.[46] The neurologic symptoms can be devastating, and may not be completely reversed once the ovarian teratomas are resected.[47]

The ultrasound appearance of cystic teratomas is, as the name suggests, predominantly cystic. The classic appearance is that of a complex cystic mass with a fat-fluid level along with an echogenic mural mass (the dermoid plug or Rokitansky nodule) (**Fig. 19**). However, varying amounts of other soft tissue components, including bone and hair, can produce varying complexity in sonographic appearance. If large amounts of calcium and fat are present, the resultant posterior acoustic shadowing may obscure the remaining mass leading to an underestimate of its size (the "tip of the iceberg" phenomenon).

Cystadenomas are uncommon in children, presenting as very large cystic masses that often fill the abdomen.[48] The serous form is more common than the mucinous type, but definitive distinction by imaging is not possible. These masses are multilocular with thin septations; solid soft-tissue components are uncommon (**Fig. 20**). The cystic epithelial carcinomas that present in adults are quite rare in children and adolescents. Cystic masses with thicker septations, internal soft tissue components, and ascites are all concerning sonographic findings for malignancy.

Solid neoplasms

Germ cell tumors are the most common malignant ovarian neoplasm in girls and include dysgerminomas, malignant teratomas, endodermal sinus tumors, embryonal carcinomas, and others.[16,35,45,49,50] Patients present with an abdominal or pelvic mass because these tumors are large at presentation (>10 cm). Pain is also a common symptom.[49] Serum tumor markers are often elevated, with alpha-fetoprotein levels increased with malignant teratomas and endodermal sinus tumors, and beta-human choriogonadotropin levels increase with embryonal carcinomas and mixed germ cell tumors.[16]

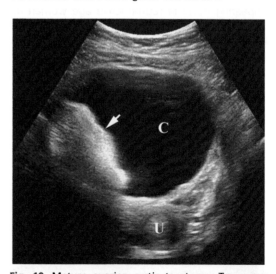

Fig. 19. Mature ovarian cystic teratoma. Transverse sonogram of a teenager with pelvic pain shows a mass that is predominantly cystic (C) anterior to the uterus (U). There is an echogenic mural nodule (*arrow*) with posterior acoustic shadowing that was shown to be mostly fat at histology.

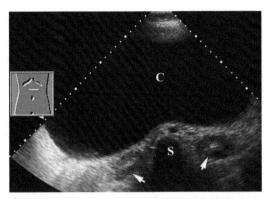

Fig. 20. Cystadenoma. Transverse sonogram in a 17-year-old girl with abdominal pain and increasing girth during the previous 6 months chows a huge uniloc-ular cystic mass (C) filling the abdomen. There were no soft tissue components and no debris within the fluid. The right ovary was not seen. Arrows point to kidneys. S, spine.

Ultrasound cannot reliably differentiate these different germ cell tumors.[35] Ultrasound shows large, predominantly solid, and complex masses with variable internal vascularity (**Fig. 21**).[51] Malig-nant teratomas are much more solid than are their benign cystic counterparts and may contain internal calcifications that are uncommon in other germ cell neoplasms. The presence of ascites, peritoneal implants, or adenopathy indicates intra-abdominal tumor dissemination.

Non–germ cell or stromal tumors account for approximately 10% of pediatric ovarian neoplasms.[50] These tumors tend to occur in

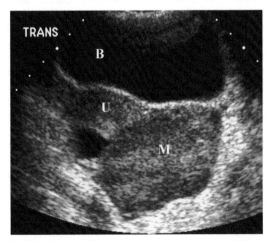

Fig. 21. Ovarian dysgerminoma. Transverse sonogram in a teenage girl with pelvic pain shows a large solid mass (M) involving the left ovary and displacing the uterus (U) to the left. A small amount of free fluid is present, but metastatic disease was not found at surgery. B, bladder.

prepubertal girls and may be hormonally active. Patients with granulosa cell tumors may present with isosexual precocious puberty from tumor production of estradiol (see **Fig. 13**).[52] As in boys, Sertoli-Leydig cell tumors in girls may produce androgens leading to virilization and premature adrenarche.[35,53] Both of these tumors have malignant potential. In the case of granulosa cell tumors, most are low stage at diagnosis and long-term survival is 97%.[52] These tumors have a variable solid and cystic appearance that is not histologically specific.

Epithelial ovarian malignancies are rare in chil-dren. Imaging findings are nonspecific.

Groin and Labia

Groin masses are uncommon in girls. A palpable labial mass in an adolescent with primary amenor-rhea may be the first indication of female pseudo-hermaphroditism, with ultrasound showing the mass to be a testis. In infants, a palpable labial mass may represent a herniated ovary (**Fig. 22**).[54] This can occur when the canal of Nuck is patent, the analog of a patent processus vaginalis in boys. An ovary is the most common structure to herniated, although hernias containing the uterus have also been reported.[55]

ACUTE PELVIS
Adnexal Torsion

Adnexal torsion occurs when there is rotation of the ovary and fallopian tube around their vascular pedicle leading to a compromise of the venous drainage and arterial supply. The dual arterial supply to the ovary may provide some protection against infarction but, depending on the degree and duration of vascular compromise, the ovary may eventually infarct. Poor fixation of the ovary predisposes to adnexal torsion, as does ovarian enlargement from cysts or tumors.[40] In younger

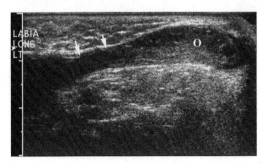

Fig. 22. Ovarian hernia. Longitudinal sonogram of the left labia in a newborn with a palpable mass shows an ovary (O) with characteristic follicles has herniated through a patent canal of Nuck (*arrows*).

patients, it is more common to have an associated ovarian lesion predisposing to torsion, but most cases in older patients are idiopathic. Only approximately 2% of patients have an associated malignancy at surgery.[56] Torsion may occur at any age, but is more common in adolescents and young adults. Patients usually present with the acute onset of pelvic pain along with nausea and vomiting, but symptoms may be more indolent. As with boys, a history of recurrent symptoms can indicate torsion and detorsion. Ovarian salvage rate is less than 50%.[57]

Because symptoms of adnexal torsion may not be distinguishable from other causes of pelvic pain, imaging is often required and ultrasound is the first and most useful test. The classic sonographic finding of ovarian torsion is an enlarged ovary at least 4 times the volume of the contralateral gonad, with hypoechoic edematous stroma and peripheral follicles (**Fig. 23**).[58,59] Ovarian size is probably the single best sonographic finding[40] and it is uncommon to have ovarian torsion when ovarian volume is less than 20 mL.[58] Larger associated cysts and masses may be present. An actual twist of the vascular pedicle may be visible.[40] The torsed ovary and fallopian tube tend to be displaced superiorly and medially, and the uterus may be deviated toward the side of torsion.[60] Isolated fallopian tube torsion has been described in adolescents and should be considered in girls with appropriate symptoms with

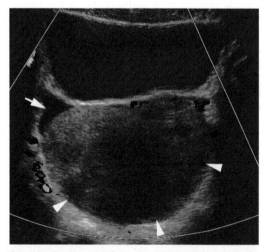

Fig. 23. Ovarian torsion. Transverse color Doppler sonogram of the pelvis in a 12-year-old girl with acute pelvic pain shows an enlarged, hypoechoic, midline left ovary with peripheral follicles (*arrowheads*), no demonstrable blood flow, and a small amount of free fluid (*arrow*). A nonsalvageable infarcted ovary was found at surgery.

a midline cystic mass and normal ipsilateral ovary.[61]

Much has been written about the lack of utility of color Doppler evaluation in adnexal torsion, and it has been repeatedly shown that a torsed ovary may still have demonstrable blood flow. However, showing that an enlarged painful ovary actually lacks blood flow is still a useful associated finding and may indicate a worse chance of ovarian salvage.[40]

Pelvic Inflammatory Disease

Ascending infection from the vagina into the upper genital tract gives rise to pelvic inflammatory disease (PID). Sexually active adolescents have the highest incidence of PID of all age groups. Sexually transmitted *Chlamydia trachomatis* and *Neisseria gonorrhoeae* are the most common causes, along with endogenous anaerobic bacteria.[26,62] Complications of PID include tubo-ovarian abscess, which occurs in 20% of adolescent patients. Long-term sequelae include infertility, chronic pelvic pain, and ectopic pregnancy.[26,62] The diagnosis is based on clinical and culture criteria, with ultrasound used to exclude complications or other unexpected diagnoses.

The ultrasound findings vary depending on the stage of the disease. Transvaginal imaging shows much greater detail than transabdominal imaging that may affect treatment decisions.[63] Mild or early disease may show no abnormality. As infection spreads, ill-definition of the uterus and ovaries from surrounding pelvic structures may occur, along with endometrial and free pelvic fluid. Progression of infection may lead to pyosalpinx, visible as fluid or debris filled dilated fallopian tubes. Further involvement may involve the ovary within a complex adnexal mass that may contain fluid and debris and will show hyperemia with color Doppler. At its most severe, intraovarian abscess may develop along with pyosalpinx to form a tubo-ovarian abscess (**Fig. 24**). Smaller abscesses usually respond well to antibiotics, but abscesses greater than 7 cm may require surgery or drainage.[64] Ultrasound allows follow-up to assess the efficacy of antibiotic therapy and can provide guidance for interventional drainage.[65]

Nongynecologic Causes

Pelvic pain may be caused by nongynecologic conditions as well. Appendicitis is the most common entity requiring emergency surgery in children and is, thus, very common. Ultrasound is an excellent method for appendicitis evaluation

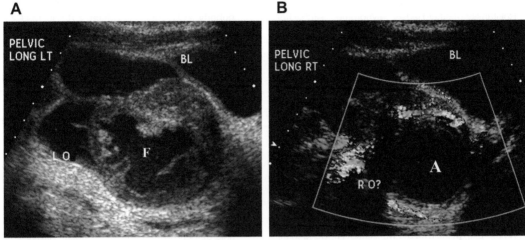

Fig. 24. Pelvic inflammatory disease complicated by tubo-ovarian abscess. (*A*) Longitudinal sonogram of the left pelvis in a teenage girl with progressive pelvic pain despite antibiotic treatment for PID shows multiple tubular, echogenic, fluid-filled structures and a dilated fimbrial end of the fallopian tube (F) indicating pyosalpinx. (*B*) Color Doppler sonogram of the right adnexa shows a right ovarian abscess (A) with peripheral hyperemia. BL, bladder; LO, left ovary; RO, right ovary.

and it is common for clinicians to ask for evaluation of both the appendix and ovaries in a girl with pelvic pain.

Less common causes of pelvic pain include intussusception in younger children, inflammatory bowel disease, and neoplasms such as Burkitt lymphoma.[66]

SUMMARY

As in adults, ultrasound is the first and often most definitive imaging modality for the evaluation of the female pelvis. An understanding of the basics of gynecologic embryology is necessary to understand congenital malformations that often underlie the reason that patients present for imaging. This allows maximization of the diagnostic potential of ultrasound, and can save these young patients from the unnecessary radiation of CT scanning and the expense (and sometimes sedation) of MR imaging.

REFERENCES

1. Ratani RS, Cohen HL, Fiore E. Pediatric gynecologic ultrasound. Ultrasound Q 2004;20:127–39.
2. Bermejo C, Martínez Ten P, Cantarero R, et al. Three-dimensional ultrasound in the diagnosis of Müllerian duct anomalies and concordance with magnetic resonance imaging. Ultrasound Obstet Gynecol 2010;35:593–601.
3. Ghi T, Casadio P, Kuleva M, et al. Accuracy of three-dimensional ultrasound in diagnosis and classification of congenital uterine anomalies. Fertil Steril 2009;92:808–13.
4. Herter LD, Golendziner E, Flores JA, et al. Ovarian and uterine sonography in healthy girls between 1 and 13 years old: correlation of findings with age and pubertal status. AJR Am J Roentgenol 2002; 178:1531–6.
5. Razzaghy-Azar M, Ghasemi F, Hallaji F, et al. Sonographic measurement of uterus and ovaries in premenarcheal healthy girls between 6 and 13 years old: correlation with age and pubertal status. J Clin Ultrasound 2011;39:64–73.
6. Garel L, Dubois J, Grignon A, et al. US of the pediatric female pelvis: a clinical perspective. Radiographics 2001;21:1393–407.
7. Troiano RN, McCarthy SM. Mullerian duct anomalies: imaging and clinical issues. Radiology 2004; 233:19–34.
8. Byrne J, Nussbaum-Blask A, Taylor WS, et al. Prevalence of Müllerian duct anomalies detected at ultrasound. Am J Med Genet 2000;94:9–12.
9. The American Fertility Society classifications of adnexal adhesions, distal tubal occlusion, tubal occlusion secondary to tubal ligation, tubal pregnancies, müllerian anomalies and intrauterine adhesions. Fertil Steril 1988;49:944–55.
10. Folch M, Pigem I, Konje JC. Mullerian agenesis: etiology, diagnosis, and management. Obstet Gynecol Surv 2000;55:644.
11. Guerrier D, Mouchel T, Pasquier L, et al. The Mayer-Rokitansky-Küster-Hauser syndrome (congenital absence of uterus and vagina)—phenotypic manifestations and genetic approaches. J Negat Results Biomed 2006;5:1.

12. Pace G, Navarra F, Paradiso GG, et al. The Mayer-Rokitansky-Küstner-Hauser syndrome. Arch Ital Urol Androl 2007;79:39–40.

13. Servaes S, Victoria T, Lovrenski J, et al. Contemporary pediatric gynecologic imaging. Semin Ultrasound CT MR 2010;31:116–40.

14. Brody JM, Koelliker SL, Frishman GN. Unicornuate uterus: imaging appearance, associated anomalies, and clinical implications. AJR Am J Roentgenol 1998;171:1341–7.

15. Junqueira BL, Allen LM, Spitzer RF, et al. Müllerian duct anomalies and mimics in children and adolescents: correlative intraoperative assessment with clinical imaging. Radiographics 2009;29:1085–103.

16. Siegel MJ. Pediatric sonography. Philadelphia: Lippincott Williams & Wilkins; 2010.

17. Ameh EA, Mshelbwala PM, Ameh N. Congenital vaginal obstruction in neonates and infants: recognition and management. J Pediatr Adolesc Gynecol 2011;24:74–8.

18. Bischoff A, Levitt MA, Breech L, et al. Hydrocolpos in cloacal malformations. J Pediatr Surg 2010;45:1241–5.

19. Blask AR, Sanders RC, Gearhart JP. Obstructed uterovaginal anomalies: demonstration with sonography. Part I. Neonates and infants. Radiology 1991;179:79.

20. Blask AR, Sanders RC, Rock JA. Obstructed uterovaginal anomalies: demonstration with sonography. Part II. Teenagers. Radiology 1991;179:84–8.

21. Chavhan GB, Parra DA, Oudjhane K, et al. Imaging of ambiguous genitalia: classification and diagnostic approach. Radiographics 2008;28:1891–904.

22. Sax L. How common is intersex? A response to Anne Fausto-Sterling. J Sex Res 2002;39(3):174–8.

23. Wright NB, Smith C, Rickwood AM, et al. Imaging children with ambiguous genitalia and intersex states. Clin Radiol 1995;50:823–9.

24. Nabhan ZM, Lee PA. Disorders of sex development. Curr Opin Obstet Gynecol 2007;19:440.

25. Zou CC, Liang L, Dong GP, et al. Peripheral precocious puberty: a retrospective study for six years in Hangzhou, China. J Paediatr Child Health 2008;44:415–8.

26. Ziereisen F, Guissard G, Damry N, et al. Sonographic imaging of the paediatric female pelvis. Eur Radiol 2005;15:1296–309.

27. Biro FM, Galvez MP, Greenspan LC, et al. Pubertal assessment method and baseline characteristics in a mixed longitudinal study of girls. Pediatrics 2010;126:e583–90.

28. Carel JC, Eugster EA, Rogol A, et al. Consensus statement on the use of gonadotropin-releasing hormone analogs in children. Pediatrics 2009;123:e752–62.

29. Mogensen SS, Aksglaede L, Mouritsen A, et al. Diagnostic work-up of 449 consecutive girls who were referred to be evaluated for precocious puberty. J Clin Endocrinol Metab 2011;96:1393–401.

30. Fahmy JL, Kaminsky CK, Kaufman F, et al. The radiological approach to precocious puberty. Br J Radiol 2000;73:560–7.

31. Stranzinger E, Strouse PJ. Ultrasound of the pediatric female pelvis. Semin Ultrasound CT MR 2008;29:98–113.

32. Deligeoroglou E, Athanasopoulos N, Tsimaris P, et al. Evaluation and management of adolescent amenorrhea. Ann N Y Acad Sci 2010;1205:23–32.

33. Dewailly D, Hieronimus S, Mirakian P, et al. Polycystic ovary syndrome (PCOS). Ann Endocrinol (Paris) 2010;71:8–13.

34. Moon LD, Brenner C, Ancliff P, et al. Non-Hodgkin's lymphoma presenting with uterine and renal enlargement in a young girl. Pediatr Radiol 2004;34:277–9.

35. Deligeoroglou E, Eleftheriades M, Shiadoes V, et al. Ovarian masses during adolescence: clinical, ultrasonographic and pathologic findings, serum tumor markers and endocrinological profile. Gynecol Endocrinol 2004;19:1–8.

36. Skiadas VT, Koutoulidis V, Eleytheriades M, et al. Ovarian masses in young adolescents: imaging findings with surgical confirmation. Eur J Gynaecol Oncol 2004;25:201–6.

37. Comparetto C, Giudici S, Coccia ME, et al. Fetal and neonatal ovarian cysts: what's their real meaning? Clin Exp Obstet Gynecol 2005;32:123–5.

38. Shimada T, Miura K, Gotoh H, et al. Management of prenatal ovarian cysts. Early Hum Dev 2008;84:417–20.

39. Levine D, Brown DL, Andreotti RF, et al. Management of asymptomatic ovarian and other adnexal cysts imaged at US: society of Radiologists in Ultrasound Consensus Conference Statement. Radiology 2010;256:943–54.

40. Chang HC, Bhatt S, Dogra VS. Pearls and pitfalls in diagnosis of ovarian torsion. Radiographics 2008;28:1355–68.

41. Amesse LS, Gibbs P, Hardy J, et al. Peritoneal inclusion cysts in adolescent females: a clinicopathological characterization of four cases. J Pediatr Adolesc Gynecol 2009;22:41–8.

42. Browne LP, Boswell HB, Crotty EJ, et al. Van Wyk and Grumbach syndrome revisited: imaging and clinical findings in pre- and postpubertal girls. Pediatr Radiol 2008;38:538–42.

43. Dovey S, Sanfilippo J. Endometriosis and the adolescent. Clin Obstet Gynecol 2010;53:420–8.

44. Van Holsbeke C, Van Calster B, Guerriero S, et al. Endometriomas: their ultrasound characteristics. Ultrasound Obstet Gynecol 2010;35:730–40.

45. Islam S, Yamout SZ, Gosche JR. Management and outcomes of ovarian masses in children and adolescents. Am Surg 2008;74:1062–5.

46. Anderson NE, Barber PA. Limbic encephalitis—a review. J Clin Neurosci 2008;15:961–71.

47. Sonn TS, Merritt DF. Anti-NMDA-receptor encephalitis: an adolescent with an ovarian teratoma. J Pediatr Adolesc Gynecol 2010;23:e141–4.

48. Barton SE, Kurek KC, Laufer MR. Recurrent bilateral serous cystadenomas in a premenarchal girl: a case report and literature review. J Pediatr Adolesc Gynecol 2010;23:e27–9.

49. Pomeranz AJ, Sabnis S. Misdiagnoses of ovarian masses in children and adolescents. Pediatr Emerg Care 2004;20:172–4.

50. Ruttenstock EM, Saxena AK, Schwinger W, et al. Pediatric ovarian tumors—dilemmas in diagnosis and management. Eur J Pediatr Surg 2010;20:116–20.

51. Guerriero S, Testa AC, Timmerman D, et al. Imaging of gynecological disease (6): clinical and ultrasound characteristics of ovarian dysgerminoma. Ultrasound Obstet Gynecol 2011;37:596–602.

52. Sivasankaran S, Itam P, Ayensu-Coker L, et al. Juvenile granulosa cell ovarian tumor: a case report and review of literature. J Pediatr Adolesc Gynecol 2009; 22:e114–7.

53. Demidov VN, Lipatenkova J, Vikhareva O, et al. Imaging of gynecological disease (2): clinical and ultrasound characteristics of Sertoli cell tumors, Sertoli-Leydig cell tumors and Leydig cell tumors. Ultrasound Obstet Gynecol 2008;31:85–91.

54. Huang CS, Luo CC, Chao HC, et al. The presentation of asymptomatic palpable movable mass in female inguinal hernia. Eur J Pediatr 2003;162: 493–5.

55. Jedrzejewski G, Stankiewicz A, Wieczorek AP. Uterus and ovary hernia of the canal of Nuck. Pediatr Radiol 2008;38:1257–8.

56. Oltmann SC, Fischer A, Barber R, et al. Pediatric ovarian malignancy presenting as ovarian torsion: incidence and relevance. J Pediatr Surg 2010;45: 135–9.

57. Anders JF, Powell EC. Urgency of evaluation and outcome of acute ovarian torsion in pediatric patients. Arch Pediatr Adolesc Med 2005;159:532–5.

58. Linam LE, Darolia R, Naffaa LN, et al. US findings of adnexal torsion in children and adolescents: size really does matter. Pediatr Radiol 2007;37:1013–9.

59. Servaes S, Zurakowski D, Laufer MR, et al. Sonographic findings of ovarian torsion in children. Pediatr Radiol 2007;37:446–51.

60. Harmon JC, Binkovitz LA, Stephens J. Uterine position in adnexal torsion: specificity and sensitivity of ipsilateral deviation of the uterus. Pediatr Radiol 2009;39:354–8.

61. Harmon JC, Binkovitz LA, Binkovitz LE. Isolated fallopian tube torsion: sonographic and CT features. Pediatr Radiol 2008;38:175–9.

62. Gray-Swain MR, Peipert JF. Pelvic inflammatory disease in adolescents. Curr Opin Obstet Gynecol 2006;18:503–10.

63. Bulas DI, Ahlstrom PA, Sivit CJ, et al. Pelvic inflammatory disease in the adolescent: comparison of transabdominal and transvaginal sonographic evaluation. Radiology 1992;183:435–9.

64. Dewitt J, Reining A, Allsworth JE, et al. Tuboovarian abscesses: is size associated with duration of hospitalization & complications? Obstet Gynecol Int 2010; 2010:847041.

65. Levenson RB, Pearson KM, Saokar A, et al. Image-guided drainage of tuboovarian abscesses of gastrointestinal or genitourinary origin: a retrospective analysis. J Vasc Interv Radiol 2011;22: 678–86.

66. Strouse PJ. Sonographic evaluation of the child with lower abdominal or pelvic pain. Radiol Clin North Am 2006;44:911–23.

Postmenopausal Endometrial Bleeding

Jean H. Lee, MD[a],*, Manjiri K. Dighe, MD[a],
Theodore J. Dubinsky, MD[a]

KEYWORDS

- Bleeding • Endometrial • Postmenopausal • Ultrasound

Endometrial bleeding is a common clinical condition in a postmenopausal woman. Postmenopausal bleeding (PMB) is defined as (1) vaginal bleeding occurring at least 12 months after complete cessation of menses in women not on hormonal replacement therapy (HRT) or (2) unpredictable vaginal bleeding occurring in postmenopausal women who have been receiving HRT for at least 12 months.[1] Although most of the postmenopausal endometrial bleeding is attributed to benign causes, including endometrial atrophy, endometrial hyperplasia, endometrial polyps, and submucosal fibroids, approximately 10% of women presenting with PMB are diagnosed with endometrial cancer.[2–4] Endometrial cancer is the most common gynecologic malignancy in United States and PMB is the common presenting symptom in 80% to 90% of patients with endometrial cancer.[4] Thus, all women presenting with PMB should be rigorously evaluated to exclude endometrial carcinoma for early diagnosis and best possible treatment because 5-year survival varies from 90% to 100% in patients with little or no myometrial involvement to 40% to 60% in patients with deep myometrial invasion.[5]

Traditionally, dilatation and curettage has been regarded as a gold standard for evaluating endometrium, which is largely replaced by an office-based endometrial biopsy (EMB). However, reported sensitivity of EMB varies from 82% to 94%, with false negative rates as high as 15%.[4,6–10] One study reported that EMB had only 43% sensitivity for detecting endometrial carcinoma.[11] The issue of access to the endometrial cavity (secondary to cervical stenosis) and sampling error may have contributed to the aforementioned variable sensitivities and false negative rates for detecting significant endometrial lesions, particularly focal lesions as opposed to the diffuse endometrial process.[4] Hysteroscopy, which allows direct visualization of the endometrial cavity, is superior in making an accurate diagnosis of focal endometrial lesions, such as endometrial polyps, submucosal fibroids, or small endometrial carcinomas. However, it is an invasive procedure that requires general anesthesia. Because of these limitations, endovaginal ultrasound is preferred as the initial study to evaluate endometrium in women with PMB.[12]

ENDOVAGINAL SONOGRAPHY
Endometrial Thickness

Endovaginal sonography is the initial imaging procedure of choice for evaluating PMB because of its ability to depict endometrial pathological conditions, its widespread availability, its excellent safety profile, and its cost-effectiveness.[12] To achieve satisfactory image quality with greater resolution, high-frequency (5.0–7.5 MHz) endovaginal probes should be used. Endometrial thickness, endometrial echotexture, margin, and the presence of abnormal vascularity within the endometrium should be thoroughly examined.[2,13] In the absence of focal endometrial abnormality, endometrial thickness has been used as an indicator for endometrial pathologic conditions with highly reproducible measurements.[14] Thus, the correct

[a] Department of Radiology, University of Washington, 1959 North East Pacific Street, Box 357115, Seattle, WA 98195, USA
* Corresponding author.
E-mail address: jeanhlee@uw.edu

Ultrasound Clin 7 (2012) 123–132
doi:10.1016/j.cult.2011.08.010
1556-858X/12/$ – see front matter © 2012 Elsevier Inc. All rights reserved.

measurement of endometrial thickness cannot be overemphasized.

The endometrial thickness should be the measurement of anterior and posterior layers of the endometrium in the sagittal plane at the level of the maximal estimated thickness (**Fig. 1**). If there is any fluid in the endometrial cavity, it should not be included. In these cases, the endometrial thickness should be the sum of 2 endometrial layers, excluding the fluid. It has been generally accepted that the cutoff for endometrial thickness is 4 or 5 mm, although some researchers advocate as thin as 3 mm.[2,4,5,12,15]

In a meta-analysis of 35 studies including 5892 postmenopausal women, using 5 mm as the upper normal limits for endometrial thickness, the sensitivity and specificity for detecting endometrial cancer were 96% (95% confidence interval [CI]: 94%–98%) and 61% (95% CI: 59%–63%). For women with PMB who have 10% pretest probability of endometrial cancer, the posttest probability decreases to 1% after negative endovaginal sonography.[16] Another published meta-analysis of 57 studies with more than 9000 patients came to a similar conclusion. The pretest probability of endometrial cancer for the overall population was 14% (95% CI: 13.3%–14.7%). Using 4 mm as the upper normal limits for endometrial thickness was associated with a posttest probability of 1.2% (95% CI: 0.4%–2.9%); and posttest probability with using 5 mm as the upper normal limits for endometrial thickness was 2.3% (95% CI: 1.2%–4.8%). A thickness more than 5 mm was associated with a posttest probability of endometrial cancer of 31.3% (95% CI: 26.1%–36.3%).[17] We have limited data on the long-term follow-up of patients with PMB, yet a study from Gull and colleagues[18] suggests safety when

a sonography-based triage is used. With at least 10 years of follow-up after PMB, no endometrial cancer was diagnosed when the endometrial thickness was less than 5 mm at the time of initial endovaginal sonography. Therefore, using the cutoff value of less than 5 mm of endometrial thickness can reasonably exclude endometrial cancer. Panel on Women's Imaging and Radiation Oncology – Gynecology from American College of Radiology (ACR) recommend using 5 mm for the cutoff of endometrial thickness.[12,13]

Women on HRT are known to have high false positive rates if the same criterion (5 mm cutoff of endometrial thickness) is used. Women on HRT had a similar sensitivity but a significantly higher false positive rate (specificity 77%; 95% CI: 75%–79%) compared with women not taking hormones (specificity 92%; 95% CI: 90%–94%) on the aforementioned meta-analysis.[16] However, an expert panel from women's imaging of the ACR Appropriateness Criteria recommends using the same criterion with the 5 mm cutoff of endometrial thickness.

Endometrial Echotexture and Morphology

Although endometrial thickness is generally accepted as the sole criterion for the sonographic evaluation of endometrium in women with PMB, the assessment of endometrial echotexture and morphology may be helpful in detecting endometrial cancer and may provide additional information. The presence of cysts in endometrium often suggests polyps, homogeneous hyperechoic endometrium suggests endometrial hyperplasia, and heterogeneous endometrium suggests endometrial cancer. However, it is not clear whether the assessment of endometrial echotexture and morphology contributes to the increase in overall diagnostic accuracy in the detection of endometrial cancer given the presence of considerable overlap of sonographic features of benign and malignant endometrial pathologic conditions.[19] In addition, the incorporation of echotexture and the morphology of endometrium to endometrial thickness decrease the sensitivity to detect endometrial cancer, although they increase the specificity and negative predictive value.[5,20] In a study of 557 women with PMB, using endometrial thickness alone (<5 mm) detected endometrial cancer with a sensitivity of 97% (95% CI: 83%–100%) and a specificity of 47% (95% CI: 42%–52%). The addition of morphologic criteria decreased the sensitivity from 97% to 77% (95% CI: 59%–90%), however, and resulted in an increase in the specificity from 47% to 84% (95% CI: 80%–87%).[5,21] Nonetheless, heterogeneous and

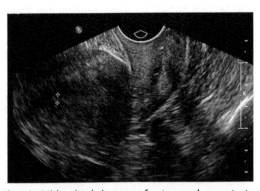

Fig. 1. Midsagittal image of uterus demonstrates smooth and homogeneous endometrium. The anterior and posterior layers of endometrial measure 3.8 mm, which is within normal limits for a postmenopausal woman.

irregular endometrium deserves further investigation with tissue sampling regardless of the endometrial thickness to exclude endometrial cancer given their high association with endometrial cancer.[4,12] In a study of 207 women with PMB, 13 of 14 cases of endometrial cancer had heterogeneous endometrium.[22]

The distinction of the focal versus diffuse endometrial process should always be made on endovaginal sonography whenever possible. Diffuse endometrial thickening is accurately diagnosed with EMB, whereas focal endometrial thickening is more accurately diagnosed with hysterosonography, direct hysteroscopic visualization, and targeted tissue sampling. Without the appropriate endovaginal sonographic evaluation, focal endometrial pathologic conditions may result in false negativity. Endovaginal ultrasound can triage the patients with PMB who would benefit from blind EMB versus hysterosonography, hysteroscopic visualization, and tissue sampling.

HYSTEROSONOGRAPHY (SALINE-INFUSION SONOHYSTEROGRAPHY)

Hysterosonography (HSG) is the imaging modality of choice if a focal intracavitary endometrial abnormality is suspected on endovaginal sonography.[12] HSG consists of the installation of sterile saline into the uterine cavity through a small catheter under endovaginal ultrasound guidance. This technique is particularly useful when (1) focal intracavitary endometrial abnormality is suspected or (2) the endometrium is not adequately delineated on endovaginal sonography. The fluid (installed sterile saline) outlining the endometrium allows better visualization, localization, and characterization of focal endometrial pathologic conditions compared with endovaginal sonography alone (**Fig. 2**A and B).[23–26] In a

study of 98 patients with PMB, HSG detected endometrial pathologic conditions with a sensitivity of 98%, a specificity of 88%, a positive predictive value of 94%, and a negative predictive value of 95%.[27] In a recent study of 70 patients with PMB, a sensitivity, a specificity, a positive predictive value, and a negative predictive value in detecting endometrial pathologic conditions by endovaginal sonography were 72.4%, 100%, 100%, and 74%, whereas those of HSG were 91.4%, 92.6%, 89.3%, and 94.1%.[26]

Hysteroscopy with direct visualization is the alternative to HSG when focal endometrial abnormality is suspected.[28] Although hysteroscopy shows similar performance characteristics compared with HSG,[29] HSG has the advantages of being less invasive, less expensive, easily achievable in an outpatient setting, and better tolerated by patients, whereas hysteroscopy generally requires an operating room setting and local or general anesthesia. Thus, it is sensible to perform HSG to confirm or better localize and characterize focal intracavitary endometrial pathologic conditions before hysteroscopy.[30] Some investigators think that HSG reduces the rate of negative hysteroscopy.[31]

HSG may be used to further evaluate the endometrium in patients with negative endovaginal sonography and biopsy with persistent bleeding given its high sensitivity in detecting small endometrial pathologic conditions. Although the risk of endometrial cancer is low in the setting of negative endovaginal sonography and biopsy, a small endometrial polyp or submucosal fibroid may account for PMB.[12] HSG may also be helpful to differentiate subendometrial cystic changes from true endometrial pathologic conditions on women with tamoxifen, which may mimic diffuse endometrial thickening on endovaginal sonography.[32]

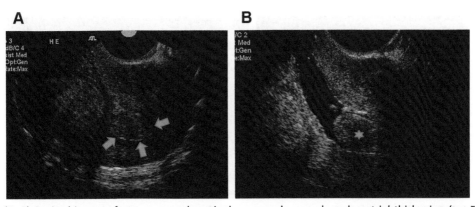

Fig. 2. (*A, B*) Sagittal image of uterus on endovaginal sonography reveals endometrial thickening (see **Fig. 2**A, *arrows*). Corresponding image of hysterosonography better demonstrates focal intracavitary lesion outlined by fluid, which confirms presence and location of focal intracavitary lesion (see **Fig. 2**B, *star*).

DOPPLER AND 3-DIMENSIONAL SONOGRAPHY

Although earlier studies demonstrated the usefulness of pulse Doppler ultrasound,[33–35] particularly resistive index (RI) in detecting endometrial carcinoma, subsequent larger series studies show significant overlap between benign and malignant endometrial pathologic conditions and fail to confirm its usefulness.[36–38] Various threshold values for RI ranging from 0.40 to 0.70 have been used to differentiate benign from malignant endometrial pathologic conditions, with most investigators recommending a threshold value of 0.40.[39,40] However, benign endometrial polyps frequently demonstrate RI values less than or equal to 0.4.[5] Therefore, RI value itself does not add additional information and is not in a routine clinical use.

However, color Doppler sonography may be of added value in further characterizing an endometrial abnormality detected at endovaginal ultrasound. For example, the presence of blood flow in focal endometrial abnormality excludes the possibility of a blood clot. The presence of a single feeding vessel in a focal endometrial abnormality may suggest an endometrial polyp, which may help in detection on endovaginal sonography.[5]

Three-dimensional (3D) sonography can be a useful adjunct to endovaginal sonography and HSG in the localization and characterization of endometrial abnormality, particularly before hysteroscopy and targeted biopsy.[12] It allows the ability to reconstruct any plane of section in orientations that cannot be obtained directly using regular, conventional endovaginal sonography and HSG (**Fig. 3**A and B). In a study by Benacerraf and colleagues,[41] 3D coronal view of the uterus was of added value to the standard 2-dimensional pelvic sonogram in 24% of all patients referred for gynecologic sonography and in up to 39% of patients with an endometrial thickness larger than 5 mm. Recently, 3D power Doppler angiography combined with 3D endovaginal sonography has been a new diagnostic tool to evaluate vascular pattern in the abnormal endometrium and endometrial volume, potentially allowing for differentiation between benign and malignant causes of a thickened endometrium.[42,43] However, many of these techniques remain in still-developing stages, and its role in a routine clinical practice has not been confirmed or validated.

CAUSES AND IMAGING FINDINGS OF PMB

Endometrial Atrophy

Endometrial atrophy is the most common cause of PMB secondary to exposure of the vessels in the underlying myometrium. In the absence of estrogen after menopause, the functional layer becomes inactive and atrophied, leaving only thin basalis layer. Atrophic endometrium on endovaginal sonography has the appearance of a thin endometrial stripe, often less than 3 mm (**Fig. 4**A and B).[2] Biopsy is insensitive in this population because tissue samples are often inadequate for diagnosis; however, the risk for endometrial cancer in this setting is very low. In case of persistent bleeding, HSG is usually the next step to exclude possible small, focal endometrial pathologic conditions.

Endometrial Hyperplasia

Endometrial hyperplasia is a common cause of PMB, which most often results from prolonged

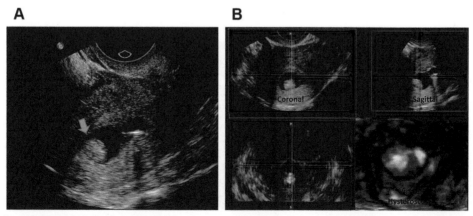

Fig. 3. (A, B) Sagittal image of uterus on hysterosonography demonstrate polypoid focal endometrial lesion (see **Fig. 3**A, *arrow*). A 3D sonography allows better localization of the focal lesion using multiplanar reconstruction (see **Fig. 3**B).

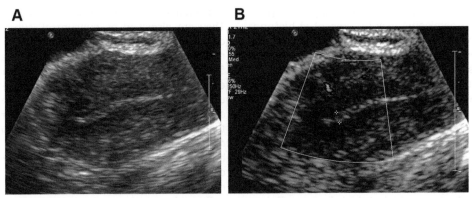

Fig. 4. (*A, B*) Sagittal image of uterus on endovaginal sonography shows thin endometrial stripe (see **Fig. 4A**) measuring 1.7 mm, without increase vascularity (see **Fig. 4B**). These imaging findings are classic for endometrial atrophy.

exposure of unopposed estrogen. Histologically, there is excessive proliferation of endometrial glands and an increased ratio of glands to stroma. Endometrial hyperplasia can further categorize as (1) hyperplasia without cellular atypia and (2) hyperplasia with cellular atypia or atypical hyperplasia.[5] Approximately a quarter of patients with atypical hyperplasia harbor coexisting foci of endometrial cancer or develop endometrial cancer in the future. The atypical hyperplasia is often focal and may be found in the background of simple hyperplasia or normal endometrium. The malignant degeneration in endometrial hyperplasia without atypia is low.

On endovaginal sonography, endometrial hyperplasia presents as a thickened endometrial stripe larger than 5 mm. The endometrium is echogenic with a well-defined margin (**Fig. 5A**). It has a similar appearance to endometrial cancer confined to the endometrium. On HSG, endometrial hyperplasia may present as focal or diffuse endometrial thickening without a localized mass

(see **Fig. 5B**).[5] At times, localized endometrial hyperplasia may mimic a sessile polyp. Identifying the feeding vessel or stalk on color Doppler ultrasound may aid in separating an endometrial polyp from localized endometrial hyperplasia. Endometrial cavity remains distensible on HSG.

Endometrial Polyp

Endometrial polyps are a localized hyperplastic overgrowth of endometrial glands and stroma around a fibrovascular core that form a sessile or pedunculated projection from the surface of endometrium.[32] They are more common in perimenopausal or postmenopausal women. Single or multiple polyps can occur ranging from a few millimeters to several centimeters in size. Although polyps are usually asymptomatic, they may result in uterine bleeding if ulceration or necrosis occurs. Patients with PMB and endometrial polyps usually undergo endometrial sampling and the removal of polyps for the following reasons: (1) to alleviate the

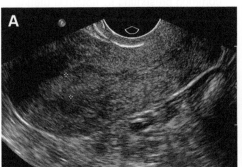

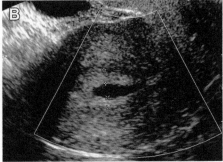

Fig. 5. (*A, B*) Sagittal image of uterus on endovaginal sonography demonstrates diffusely thickened endometrium that measures 8.7 mm (see **Fig. 5A**). Corresponding HSG image with color Doppler reveals diffusely thickened endometrium with no vascularity, which is consistent with endometrial hyperplasia (see **Fig. 5B**).

symptoms of bleeding, (2) foci of atypical hyperplasia or carcinoma may be present at histopathology in a benign-seeming polyp, and (3) endometrial polyps and carcinoma may coexist in the same patient.[5,44]

The sonographic appearance of polyps can be variable. They may present as focal or diffuse endometrial thickening. When focal, they are typically round, hyperechoic masses within the endometrial cavity. Small cystic areas corresponding to dilated glands filled with proteinaceous fluid may also be seen within the polyps (**Fig. 6**).[32] Although not necessary for diagnosis, cystic areas are fairly specific for benign endometrial disease.[2] Polyps presenting as diffuse endometrial thickening are difficult to diagnose secondary to the presence of considerable imaging overlap with endometrial hyperplasia (**Fig. 7**A). The presence of a feeding artery on color Doppler sonography in suspected endometrial pathologic conditions may favor an endometrial polyp over other pathologic conditions, including submucosal fibroid or endometrial hyperplasia (see **Fig. 7**B). Polyps are better visualized on HSG. With HSG, polyps present as echogenic, smooth, intracavitary masses outlined by fluid that demonstrate no interruption of the endometrial lining (see **Fig. 7**C).

Leiomyoma

Leiomyomas, commonly known as fibroids, are benign neoplastic growths of smooth muscle cells within the myometrium. They occur in up to 40% of women aged older than 35 years and are seen on 75% of hysterectomy specimens.[2] Leiomyomas are not encapsulated but contain a pseudocapsule

representing compressed adjacent myometrium. They are classified as subserosal, submucosal, or intramural based on their locations. Leiomyomas are classified as submucosal when at least 50% of the lesion protrudes into the endometrial cavity. Submucosal leiomyomas may result in uterine bleeding caused by congestion, necrosis, and ulceration of their surface or just by increasing the surface area of the endometrial cavity and disrupting the normal sloughing process.[5] These benign leiomyomas regress with estrogen withdrawal as seen in postmenopausal women. Malignant degeneration is rare.

On endovaginal sonography, submucosal leiomyomas are typically hypoechoic, well-defined, solid masses, with an overlying layer of echogenic endometrium (**Fig. 8**A). They often distort the interface between the endometrium and myometrium and show acoustic attenuation, which often results in poor visualization of the endometrium. Submucosal leiomyomas are sometimes larger than polyps and may demonstrate multiple feeding vessels on color Doppler sonography. They may demonstrate calcifications. The most important sonographic feature to differentiate the submucosal leiomyomas from polyps is to ascertain the location of the endometrial lining with regard to the lesion.[32] On HSG, the relationship between the endometrial lining and a suspected endometrial lesion can be better evaluated because the endometrial lining is well outlined by the installation of normal saline (see **Fig. 8**B). HSG is particularly useful if the endometrium is poorly visualized secondary to the distortion of the endometrial cavity, acoustic attenuation, and calcification in combination with the atrophic endometrium in women with PMB.

Endometrial Cancer

Endometrial cancer is the most common malignancy of the female genital tract. The most common presenting symptom is uterine bleeding. Approximately 90% of endometrial cancer is adenocarcinomas. Other histologic subsets include squamous cell carcinoma, papillary, and clear cell carcinoma. The disease is surgically staged. The mainstay of treatment is surgical staging, with hysterectomy and lymph node dissection as indicated.[2]

The sonographic appearance of endometrial carcinoma is variable. The most common appearance is nonspecific thickening, which significantly overlaps with endometrial hyperplasia. Endometrial carcinomas may present as (1) diffuse endometrial thickening, hyperechoic with well-defined borders (**Fig. 9**A); (2) endometrial thickening with

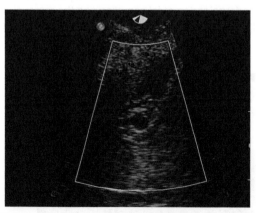

Fig. 6. Biopsy confirmed endometrial polyp. Sagittal image of uterus on endovaginal ultrasound with color Doppler demonstrates localized thickening of endometrium with multiple cystic spaces. No vascularity was present.

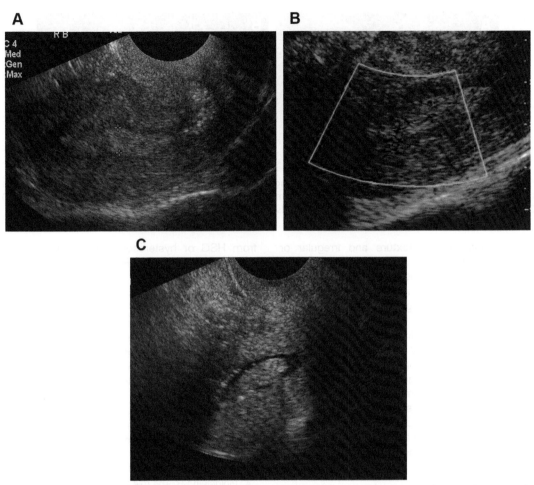

Fig. 7. (*A, B, C*) Biopsy confirmed endometrial polyp. Sagittal image of uterus on endovaginal sonography demonstrate diffuse thickening of endometrium (see **Fig. 7A**). Color Doppler image reveals vascular stalk (see **Fig. 7B**). Hysterosonography shows smooth, echogenic polypoid mass without interruption of overlying endometrium, consistent with endometrial polyp (see **Fig. 7C**).

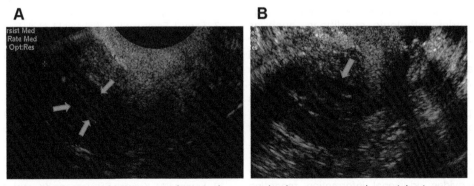

Fig. 8. (*A, B*) Sagittal image of uterus on endovaginal sonography demonstrates endometrial stripe measuring 8.5 mm. Endometrium appear homogeneously hypoechoic (*blue arrows*, **Fig. 8A**). Corresponding HSG image better visualize the hypoechoic mass with well-defined border and broad base (*blue arrow*), which was proven as submucosal leiomyoma (**Fig. 8B**).

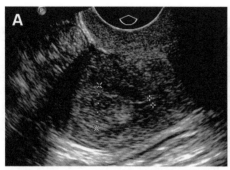
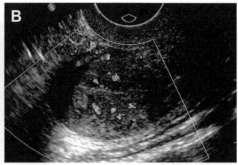

Fig. 9. (*A, B*) Biopsy confirmed endometrial cancer. Sagittal image of uterus on endovaginal sonography demonstrates diffuse endometrial thickening measuring 13 mm. The thickened endometrium is echogenic (see **Fig. 9**A). Color Doppler images reveals multiple feeding vessels within the thickened endometrium (see **Fig. 9**B).

a heterogeneous echotexture and irregular or poorly defined margins; and (3) a heterogeneous masslike lesion.[5] On HSG, endometrial cancer is suspected when there is a single layer thicker than 8 mm that is irregular, broad-based, and poorly marginated or when the endometrial-myometrial interface is disrupted.[32] Poor distensibility of the uterine cavity is reported to be a useful sign for diagnosing endometrial carcinoma.[27,45]

On color Doppler imaging, endometrial cancers typically demonstrate multiple feeding vessels and show moderate vascularity (see **Fig. 9**B).[21] However, stalk flow may be seen in polypoid endometrial carcinomas. The presence of hypovascularity does not exclude endometrial carcinoma.

SUMMARY

Endovaginal sonography is a powerful initial diagnostic tool to evaluate endometrial pathologic conditions in women with PMB. Endovaginal sonography is highly sensitive to detect endometrial cancer and reasonably excludes endometrial cancer if endometrial thickness is less than 5 mm. Because most PMB is attributed to benign endometrial pathologic conditions, such as endometrial hyperplasia, endometrial polyps, or submucosal leiomyomas, normal endometrial thickness with homogeneous echotexture may prevent an unnecessary and inappropriate procedure. However, endovaginal sonography does not replace definitive histopathologic diagnosis, therefore, abnormal echotexture and morphology of the endometrium warrants further evaluation, including HSG, hysteroscopy, EMB, and histopathologic examination. Endovaginal sonography also provides additional information regarding the focal versus diffuse process in the setting of endometrial pathologic conditions, which allows the identification of patients who would benefit

from HSG or hysterosonography from patients who would benefit from EMB.

REFERENCES

1. Albers JR, Hull SK, Wesley RM. Abnormal uterine bleeding. Am Fam Physician 2004;69:1915–26.
2. Davidson KG, Dubinsky TJ. Ultrasonographic evaluation of the endometrium in postmenopausal vaginal bleeding. Radiol Clin North Am 2003;41:769–80.
3. Karlsson B, Granberg S, Hellberg P, et al. Comparative study of transvaginal sonography and hysteroscopy for the detection of pathologic endometrial lesions in women with postmenopausal bleeding. J Ultrasound Med 1994;13:757–62.
4. Goldstein SR. The role of transvaginal ultrasound or endometrial biopsy in the evaluation of the menopausal endometrium. Am J Obstet Gynecol 2009; 201:5–11.
5. Reinhold C, Khalili I. Postmenopausal bleeding: value of imaging. Radiol Clin North Am 2002;40: 527–62.
6. Zorlu CG, Cobanoglu O, Isik AZ, et al. Accuracy of pipelle endometrial sampling in endometrial carcinoma. Gynecol Obstet Invest 1994;38:272–5.
7. Ferry J, Farnsworth A, Webster M, et al. The efficacy of the pipelle endometrial biopsy in detecting endometrial carcinoma. Aust N Z J Obstet Gynaecol 1993;33:76–8.
8. Guido RS, Kanbour-Shakir A, Rulin MC, et al. Pipelle endometrial sampling. Sensitivity in the detection of endometrial cancer. J Reprod Med 1995;40:553–5.
9. Goldchmit R, Katz Z, Blickstein I, et al. The accuracy of endometrial pipelle sampling with and without sonographic measurement of endometrial thickness. Obstet Gynecol 1993;82:727–30.
10. Larson DM, Krawisz BR, Johnson KK, et al. Comparison of the Z-sampler and Novak endometrial biopsy instruments for in-office diagnosis of endometrial cancer. Gynecol Oncol 1994;54:64–7.

11. Stovall TG, Solomon SK, Ling FW. Endometrial sampling prior to hysterectomy. Obstet Gynecol 1989;73:405–9.

12. Bennett GL, Andreotti RF, Lee SI, et al. ACR appropriateness criteria(®) on abnormal vaginal bleeding. J Am Coll Radiol 2011;8:460–8.

13. Goldstein RB, Bree RL, Benson CB, et al. Evaluation of the woman with postmenopausal bleeding: society of radiologists in ultrasound-sponsored consensus conference statement. J Ultrasound Med 2001;20:1025–36.

14. Delisle MF, Villeneuve M, Boulvain M. Measurement of endometrial thickness with transvaginal ultrasonography: is it reproducible? J Ultrasound Med 1998;17:481–4 [quiz: 5–6].

15. van Hanegem N, Breijer MC, Khan KS, et al. Diagnostic evaluation of the endometrium in postmenopausal bleeding: an evidence-based approach. Maturitas 2011;68:155–64.

16. Smith-Bindman R, Kerlikowske K, Feldstein VA, et al. Endovaginal ultrasound to exclude endometrial cancer and other endometrial abnormalities. JAMA 1998;280:1510–7.

17. Gupta JK, Chien PF, Voit D, et al. Ultrasonographic endometrial thickness for diagnosing endometrial pathology in women with postmenopausal bleeding: a meta-analysis. Acta Obstet Gynecol Scand 2002; 81:799–816.

18. Gull B, Karlsson B, Milsom I, et al. Can ultrasound replace dilation and curettage? A longitudinal evaluation of postmenopausal bleeding and transvaginal sonographic measurement of the endometrium as predictors of endometrial cancer. Am J Obstet Gynecol 2003;188:401–8.

19. Hulka CA, Hall DA, McCarthy K, et al. Endometrial polyps, hyperplasia, and carcinoma in postmenopausal women: differentiation with endovaginal sonography. Radiology 1994;191:755–8.

20. Hanggi W, Brandenberger AW, Ammann M, et al. Diagnosis of malignant uterine tumors by transvaginal ultrasound. Ultraschall Med 1995;16:2–7 [in German].

21. Reinhold C. The use of endovaginal sonography and Doppler ultrasound in detection of endometrial carcinoma in women presenting with postmenopausal bleeding [master's thesis] [Master's thesis]. Montreal (Canada): MaGill University; 1999.

22. Sheikh M, Sawhney S, Khurana A, et al. Alteration of sonographic texture of the endometrium in postmenopausal bleeding. A guide to further management. Acta Obstet Gynecol Scand 2000;79:1006–10.

23. Cullinan JA, Fleischer AC, Kepple DM, et al. Sonohysterography: a technique for endometrial evaluation. Radiographics 1995;15:501–14 [discussion: 15–6].

24. Dubinsky TJ, Stroehlein K, Abu-Ghazzeh Y, et al. Prediction of benign and malignant endometrial disease: hysterosonographic-pathologic correlation. Radiology 1999;210:393–7.

25. Williams CD, Marshburn PB. A prospective study of transvaginal hydrosonography in the evaluation of abnormal uterine bleeding. Am J Obstet Gynecol 1998;179:292–8.

26. Mathew M, Gowri V, Rizvi SG. Saline infusion sonohysterography - an effective tool for evaluation of the endometrial cavity in women with abnormal uterine bleeding. Acta Obstet Gynecol Scand 2010;89:140–2.

27. Bree RL, Bowerman RA, Bohm-Velez M, et al. US evaluation of the uterus in patients with postmenopausal bleeding: a positive effect on diagnostic decision making. Radiology 2000;216:260–4.

28. Lee SI. An imaging algorithm for evaluation of abnormal uterine bleeding: does sonohysterography play a role? Menopause 2007;14:823–5.

29. van Dongen H, de Kroon CD, Jacobi CE, et al. Diagnostic hysteroscopy in abnormal uterine bleeding: a systematic review and meta-analysis. BJOG 2007;114:664–75.

30. Bignardi T, Van den Bosch T, Condous G. Abnormal uterine and post-menopausal bleeding in the acute gynaecology unit. Best Pract Res Clin Obstet Gynaecol 2009;23:595–607.

31. Erdem M, Bilgin U, Bozkurt N, et al. Comparison of transvaginal ultrasonography and saline infusion sonohysterography in evaluating the endometrial cavity in pre- and postmenopausal women with abnormal uterine bleeding. Menopause 2007;14: 846–52.

32. Shi AA, Lee SI. Radiological reasoning: algorithmic workup of abnormal vaginal bleeding with endovaginal sonography and sonohysterography. AJR Am J Roentgenol 2008;191:S68–73.

33. Bourne TH, Campbell S, Steer CV, et al. Detection of endometrial cancer by transvaginal ultrasonography with color flow imaging and blood flow analysis: a preliminary report. Gynecol Oncol 1991;40:253–9.

34. Bourne TH, Campbell S, Whitehead MI, et al. Detection of endometrial cancer in postmenopausal women by transvaginal ultrasonography and colour flow imaging. BMJ 1990;301:369.

35. Merce LT, Lopez Garcia G, de la Fuente F. Doppler ultrasound assessment of endometrial pathology. Acta Obstet Gynecol Scand 1991;70:525–30.

36. Conoscenti G, Meir YJ, Fischer-Tamaro L, et al. Endometrial assessment by transvaginal sonography and histological findings after D & C in women with postmenopausal bleeding. Ultrasound Obstet Gynecol 1995;6:108–15.

37. Chan FY, Chau MT, Pun TC, et al. Limitations of transvaginal sonography and color Doppler imaging in the differentiation of endometrial carcinoma from benign lesions. J Ultrasound Med 1994;13:623–8.

38. Flam F, Almstrom H, Hellstrom AC, et al. Value of uterine artery Doppler in endometrial cancer. Acta Oncol 1995;34:779–82.

39. Hata T, Hata K, Senoh D, et al. Doppler ultrasound assessment of tumor vascularity in gynecologic disorders. J Ultrasound Med 1989;8:309–14.

40. Kurjak A, Shalan H, Kupesic S, et al. An attempt to screen asymptomatic women for ovarian and endometrial cancer with transvaginal color and pulsed Doppler sonography. J Ultrasound Med 1994;13:295–301.

41. Benacerraf BR, Shipp TD, Bromley B. Which patients benefit from a 3D reconstructed coronal view of the uterus added to standard routine 2D pelvic sonography? AJR Am J Roentgenol 2008;190:626–9.

42. Alcazar JL, Galvan R. Three-dimensional power Doppler ultrasound scanning for the prediction of endometrial cancer in women with postmenopausal bleeding and thickened endometrium. Am J Obstet Gynecol 2009;200:44.e1–6.

43. Odeh M, Vainerovsky I, Grinin V, et al. Three-dimensional endometrial volume and 3-dimensional power Doppler analysis in predicting endometrial carcinoma and hyperplasia. Gynecol Oncol 2007;106:348–53.

44. Dubinsky TJ, Parvey HR, Gormaz G, et al. Transvaginal hysterosonography: comparison with biopsy in the evaluation of postmenopausal bleeding. J Ultrasound Med 1995;14:887–93.

45. Laifer-Narin SL, Ragavendra N, Lu DS, et al. Transvaginal saline hysterosonography: characteristics distinguishing malignant and various benign conditions. AJR Am J Roentgenol 1999;172:1513–20.

Pelvic Pain: Ultrasound of the Bowel

Caitlin T. McGregor, MD, FRCP

KEYWORDS

- Ultrasound • Bowel • Appendicitis • Diverticulitis
- Crohn's disease • Pelvis

RIGHT LOWER QUADRANT PAIN: GASTROINTESTINAL ULTRASOUND

Ultrasound (US) is a useful modality for women of reproductive age presenting with acute or chronic lower quadrant pain. It is superior to CT for the evaluation of the uterus and ovaries, does not involve radiation, and is widely available. The most recent American College of Radiology Appropriateness Criteria for acute pelvic pain in the reproductive age group states that transvaginal US should be used as the initial test when obstetric or gynecologic etiologies are suspected.[1] In the setting of a negative β-hCG result and a clinical suspicion of gastrointestinal (GI) or genitourinary disease, a CT scan is a useful first test.[1] Clinical diagnosis, however, can be especially challenging in reproductive women because gynecologic causes, such as tubo-ovarian abscess, ruptured ovarian cyst, and ovarian torsion, can have a similar presentation to GI tract disease. Pelvic pain, fever, nausea, vomiting, and an elevated white count are nonspecific. When a uterine or ovarian cause for a patient's symptoms is not found on US, a systematic search must be performed for nongynecologic causes, including diseases of the bowel. Correctly diagnosing both gynecologic and nongynecologic causes of pelvic pain on US allows appropriate triaging and correct initiation of medical versus surgical therapy. This avoids unnecessary radiation and laparotomy. An understanding of both transabdominal and transvaginal sonography of the GI tract is, therefore, essential in performing a complete pelvic evaluation of premenopausal women presenting to the US department with pelvic pain. This article includes a review of the anatomy of the GI tract and bowel wall in addition to the techniques used to perform a thorough evaluation of the bowel with US. GI causes of pelvic pain are then discussed, including appendicitis, diverticulitis, inflammatory bowel disease, epiploic appendagitis, omental infarction, and infection.

ANATOMY

The stratified appearance of the normal bowel wall on US reflects its histologic construction (**Fig. 1**). The innermost echogenic line corresponds to the interface between the mucosa and the lumen. The next concentric hypoechoic ring is the muscularis mucosa, followed by the echogenic submucosa and finally by the outermost hypoechoic muscularis propria. Histologically this muscular layer is composed of a longitudinal layer and a circular layer; however, these 2 layers are not resolved on US. The serosa is the outermost thin echogenic line but is not always visible because it blends in with the adjacent echogenic fat. This concentric arrangement is constant throughout the GI tract from the esophagus to the rectum, including the appendix. Of CT, MR imaging, and US, US is the only modality to resolve all 5 layers, which makes it particularly useful in evaluating the bowel.

Understanding the mesenteric attachments is important when evaluating the bowel by any modality. On US, knowledge of which segments are fixed in position and which segments are mobile aids in localizing the segment of interest. A mesentery is a double layer of visceral peritoneum that wraps around a segment of bowel and attaches it to the posterior abdominal wall. The small bowel mesentery attaches along the posterior abdominal wall in a line from the left side of L2 downwards and rightwards toward the

The author has nothing to disclose.
Division of Abdominal Imaging, Department of Medical Imaging, Sunnybrook Health Sciences Centre, University of Toronto, 2075 Bayview Avenue, Toronto, ON M4N 3M5, Canada
E-mail address: caitlin.mcgregor@sunnybrook.ca

Ultrasound Clin 7 (2012) 133–153
doi:10.1016/j.cult.2011.11.003

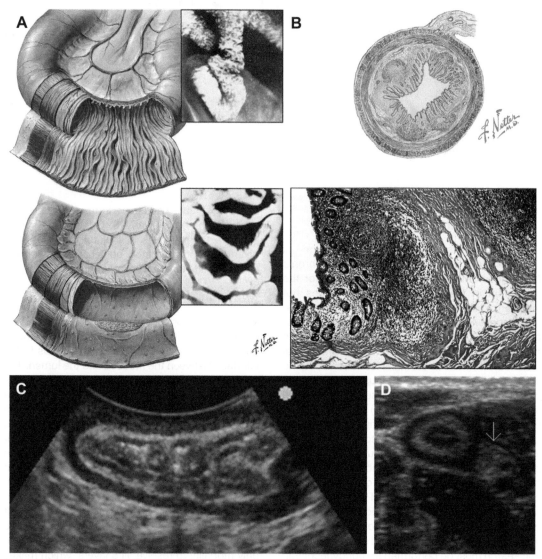

Fig. 1. (A) Netter diagram illustrating the layers of the bowel wall. (*upper panel*) Jejeunum with correlation on a barium study, (*lower panel*) ileum with correlation on a barium study. (B) Netter diagram illustrating the histologic arrangement of the bowel wall layers; shown both as a schematic (*upper illustration*) and on a histologic specimen (*lower illustration*). (C) US image of the normal stomach in cross section demonstrating the concentric echogenic and hypoechoic rings. (D) Abnormal appendix in cross section demonstrating the rings and adjacent mesoappendix (*white arrow*). ([A, B] Netter illustration from www.netterimages.com. © Elsevier, Inc. All rights reserved.)

right sacroiliac joint. This is the root of the small bowel mesentery. The superior mesenteric artery and superior mesenteric vein run between the 2 layers of peritoneum entering at the root. This posterior line of attachment is short but fans out to the free edge of the small bowel mesentery where the small bowel is located. The free edge of the small bowel mesentery is, therefore, essentially the length of the entire small bowel (approximately 6 m). This allows the small bowel to be mobile, making it difficult on US to be precise about location along the small bowel.

The cecum is the segment of large bowel inferior to the ileocecal valve. This valve is a landmark on US. The cecum does not have its own mesentery and has a variable attachment to the posterior abdominal wall. This accounts for the anatomic variability in position and mobility of the cecum observed in normal individuals (**Fig. 2**). This is an important point to understand when trying the find the cecum, terminal ileum, and appendix on US.

The appendix arises from the cecum posteromedial to the ileocecal valve and approximately 2.5 cm inferior. The length of the appendix is

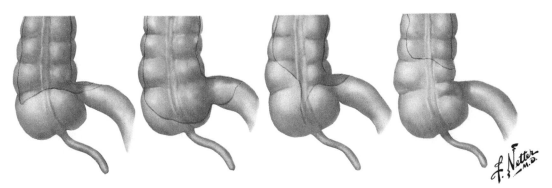

Fig. 2. Netter illustrations showing the variable posterior attachment of the cecum (*shaded area*). (Netter illustration from www.netterimages.com. © Elsevier, Inc. All rights reserved.)

variable (2–5 cm). Although the relationship of the origin of the appendix to the ileocecal valve is fixed, the tip of the appendix is variable. The origin of the appendix lacks a valve. This is a key feature in differentiating it from the terminal ileum on US (**Fig. 3**). The appendix has its own mesentery, called the mesoappendix. Like the small bowel, the appendix lies along the free edge of the

mesoappendix; however, unlike the small bowel, the mesoappendix does not attach to the posterior abdominal wall but to the edge of the small bowel mesentery (**Fig. 4**).

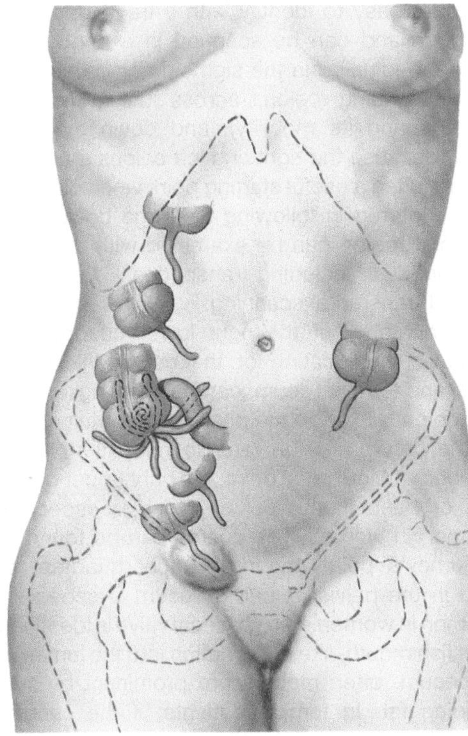

The right colon is covered by peritoneum anteriorly and laterally, which then attaches it to the posterior abdominal wall. The right colon is fixed in position and is considered a retroperitoneal organ. This arrangement is true for the left colon as well.

The transverse colon is suspended in its own mesentery, called the transverse mesocolon, which then attaches to the posterior abdominal wall similar to the small bowel mesentery. The posterior attachment or root is in a horizontal line beginning over the second portion of the duodenum extending above the pancreatic head and then along the inferior border of the pancreatic body and tail. The length of the transverse mesocolon is variable so that the transverse colon is also variable in position and can extend directly across the upper abdomen or can dip deep into the pelvis. The transverse mesocolon effectively divides the abdomen into a supracolic compartment and an infracolic compartment.

The sigmoid is also a suspended segment of bowel. Its mesentery can be thought of in 2 segments. The superior segment arises from the descending colon mesocolon and attaches along the medial side of the left iliac vessels. The inferior part has its root along the third sacral vertebra. This relationship causes the root of the sigmoid mesentery to attach to the pelvic sidewall in the configuration of an inverted V. Again this allows mobility so that the sigmoid can extend over to the right lower quadrant and cause right lower quadrant pain.

Finally the rectum is an extraperitoneal structure, fixed in location. Peritoneum covers the rectum along the mid and upper thirds of the anterior wall and around the upper third of the lateral walls (**Box 1**).

Fig. 3. Netter illustrations showing the variable position of both the appendix and the cecum. The constant relationship of the cecum, ileocecal valve, and appendix is important to understand when attempting to find these structures on US. (Netter illustration from www.netterimages.com. © Elsevier, Inc. All rights reserved.)

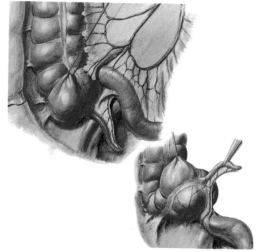

Fig. 4. Netter illustration showing the anatomy of the mesoappendix. (Netter illustration from www.netter images.com. © Elsevier, Inc. All rights reserved.)

TECHNIQUE

Any US examination of the female pelvis should begin with noncompressive transabdominal scanning with a 3.5-MHz or 5-MHz curvilinear probe to gain a panoramic view of the pelvis. A higher frequency curvilinear probe can be advantageous in thinner patients. A distended bladder is helpful in evaluating the mid to distal sigmoid and the rectum transabdominally.[2] Examination of the bowel should then continue with a high-frequency linear probe. In thinner patients, a linear 12-MHz probe can produce exquisite images. Often alternating between multiple probes is necessary.

It is advantageous to have patients fast for at least 4 hours in subacute or chronic presentations, and often fasting is self-imposed in acute patients. Bowel gas is cited as a limitation of bowel US; however, in practice, diseased segments are often gasless. Graded compression and moving a patient into multiple positions can displace gas from the field of view.

Box 1	
Fixation of the bowel by segment	
Intraperitoneal and mobile	Small bowel Appendix Cecum Transverse colon Sigmoid colon
Extraperitoneal and fixed	Duodenum—second and third portions Right colon Left colon Rectum

The graded compression technique was first described by Puylaert in 1986 to evaluate the appendix.[3] It is now widely applied to sonography of the GI tract. The purpose of graded compression is 3-fold: to reduce the distance between the transducer and the bowel segment of interest; to displace bowel gas, improving visibility; and to minimize tenderness and discomfort. Graded compression consists of slowly and steadily compressing the bowel between the anterior abdominal wall and the posterior abdominal wall. In larger patients, performing additional compression by placing the left hand beneath a patient and pushing toward the transducer can improve visualization.[4] Positioning patients in the left lateral decubitus position helps identify a retrocecal appendix. Turning patients in multiple directions can be used in an effort to get air to move out of the field of view.

Bowel presets entered by manufacturers are now in general use and often include compound imaging. Harmonic imaging is useful when scanning the bowel due to the highly reflective nature of air. The use of more than one focal zone is also suggested.

The first task is to identify the anatomy of the GI tract. Often the sigmoid, left, transverse, and right colon are easy to identify with a transabdominal approach and can be scanned in a contiguous fashion, beginning in the sigmoid and moving up the descending colon, across the transverse (remembering its mobility), and down the right colon. Because the right and left colons are fixed, they are often a useful starting point when difficulty is encountered in following the large bowel. The anorectal region can be examined with a variety of techniques, including transperineal, transvaginal, and transrectal scanning.

The anatomy of the right lower quadrant, in particular the location of the cecum, ileocecal valve, and terminal ileum, can be challenging. The right colon is fixed to the posterior abdominal wall but the cecum may be variable in location. It can be found at McBurney point, the right upper quadrant, or deep in the pelvis, which is especially common in women. The cecum can be found at McBurney's point, the right upper quadrant or deep in the pelvis. A pelvic cecum is especially common in women. The ileocecal valve is identified by its fish mouth–like invagination into the lumen of the cecum, often made more prominent by surrounding fat. In female patients, if the cecum, terminal ileum, and appendix are not seen transabdominally, a transvaginal US must be performed.

Other than the terminal ileum and duodenum, the small bowel is difficult to precisely localize on US and generally topographic criteria are used: the jejunum in the left upper quadrant and the ileum in the pelvis. As discussed previously, the small bowel mesentery allows great mobility so that topographic criteria are not always correct. small bowel mesentery allows great mobility and this is not always the case. The jejunum is characterized by many valvulae conniventes whereas the ileum has far fewer.

Hydrocolosonography is described in the literature mainly in the setting of inflammatory bowel disease.[5] It consists of administrating a water enema and buscopan after bowel preparation; however, this has not become part of routine clinical practice. Giving oral water at the time of the scan can greatly aid in visualization of the stomach and duodenum. Oral polyethylene glycol (PEG) has also been proposed for studying the small bowel with US. Like hydrocolosonography it has been described mostly in the setting of inflammatory bowel disease and has not become part of routine clinical practice.[6]

Although there is some variation in the literature, most investigators use a cutoff of 4 mm to identify a thickened bowel wall. Wall thickness is usually measured in the transverse plane from the inner echogenic line to the outer edge of the serosal surface. If a bowel segment is determined to be thickened then the layers must be carefully analyzed. If the bowel wall layers are preserved, a malignant process is considered unlikely.[7] Conversely, if the layers are destroyed, both malignancy and severe inflammation (common in Crohn's disease) are possible.

When the layers are thickened but preserved, determining which layer is the most involved can provide additional information. An epicenter of thickening that is the submucosal layer and which is circumferential and echogenic indicates an acute nonmalignant process intrinsic to that loop of bowel (**Fig. 5**A).[8] A thickened outer layer, especially if located on one side of the bowel only, is more likely secondary to an adjacent inflammatory process (see **Fig. 5**B). This finding is helpful in avoiding potential pitfalls, such as diagnosing cecal disease, when thickening is secondary to adjacent appendicitis.

US is a real-time technique and an assessment of peristalsis and of the compressibility of the bowel should also be made. The luminal content should also be evaluated: empty, fluid filled, stool filled, or air filled (in which case the posterior wall is obscured unless the air is displaced with compression or by turning the patient). The real-time advantage of US also allows localization of the point of maximum tenderness.

APPENDICITIS

Appendicitis is the most common cause for emergency surgery in the Western world.[9] It is known that preoperative imaging lowers the negative laparotomy rate and this is especially true for women.[10] A recent meta-analysis of the diagnostic performance of US versus CT revealed a sensitivity of 78% for US and 91% for CT with specificity of 83% for US and 90% for CT.[11]

There are a variety of management options in appendicitis, including laparotomy, laparoscopy, and conservative treatment with antibiotics plus or minus percutaneous drainage. In combination with the clinical presentation, surgeons require staging of appendicitis on imaging to make management decisions. The degree of periappendiceal inflammation; the degree of cecal or adjacent small bowel thickening; the presence of focal collections, free air, bowel obstruction, or ileus; and mesenteric seeding should be evaluated.

In order to identify the appendix, the graded compression technique should be used beginning

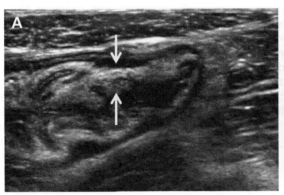
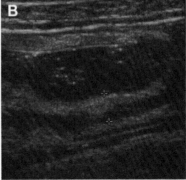

Fig. 5. (*A*) Marked thickening of the echogenic submucosal layer (*between arrows*) indicative of acute inflammation in this patient with infectious colitis. (*B*) Asymmetric thickening of the posterior wall (*between calipers*) of the cecum involving the outer layers more than the inner layers—in this patient, secondary thickening of the cecum is due to adjacent appendicitis.

in the right upper quadrant just below the liver (**Boxes 2** and **3**). Once the ileocecal valve and terminal ileum are identified, the appendix should be seen arising from the cecum without a valve. Because a retrocecal appendix is common, when the appendix is not seen, patients should be placed in a left lateral decubitus position (**Fig. 6**). All women should receive a transvaginal examination if the appendix is not seen from above. By identifying the ileocecal valve and the origin of the appendix separately, a common pitfall of mistaking the terminal ileum for the appendix or vice versa is avoided. Once the origin of the appendix is seen, then scanning commences along the entire length of appendix to prove it is blind ending, aperistaltic, and with gut signature. This avoids mistaking a loop of bowel as the appendix and other potential pitfalls, such as a dilated ureter, fallopian tube, or vessel (**Table 1**). It also ensures that inflammation limited to the tip, so-called tip appendicitis, is not overlooked.

Once an appendix is correctly localized, the next question is to determine if it is normal or abnormal.

One of the most established criteria for diagnosing appendicitis on US is an outer diameter under compression of 6 mm. This sign is more useful in excluding appendicitis; that is, an appendix measuring 6 mm or less is highly unlikely to be acutely inflamed. When an appendix measures more than 6 mm, additional signs should be used to rule in appendicitis.[12] The one exception to this is in cases of a perforated appendix that has deflated, producing a measurement less than 6 mm. The periappendiceal changes in these cases should prevent this pitfall. Another useful sign in ruling out appendicitis is demonstrating that the appendix is ovoid in cross section; care must be taken to ensure that this is the case along the entire length of the appendix.[13] When inflamed, the appendix is almost always round in cross section. This is in contrast to a loop of bowel, which maintains its ovoid cross section even when abnormal. If bowel wall thickening is noted in a segment with an ovoid cross section, an abnormal appendix is unlikely. If an appendix is compressible along its entire length, appendicitis is also reliably ruled out.[14]

Tenderness over the appendix is useful; however, this finding is not entirely specific for

---

Box 3
Signs to rule in appendicitis

Single wall thickness greater than 3 mm

Noncompressible

Presence of Doppler signal

Loss or irregularity of the submucosal layer

Focal tenderness

---

appendicitis (for example, when there is terminal ileitis) and can also be absent particularly in the elderly or very young and when a patient is on steroids or otherwise immunosuppressed.

Once an appendix is found to measure more than 6 mm and noncompressible, a careful assessment of the appendicular wall and content must be performed. If the diameter of the appendix is greater than 6 mm, it is suggested that measuring individual wall thickness as greater than 3 mm can increase confidence that the appendix is inflamed. This is helpful in situations when a normal appendix measures more than 6 mm because of inspisated fecal content. In many cases of appendicitis, however, the wall is thinned rather than thickened, meaning that 3 mm is useful to rule in inflammation but not to rule it out. Another helpful tool in avoiding this potential false-positive result is to examine the content. A noncompressible appendix filled with fluid is concerning. In contrast, inspisated fecal content is echogenic and noncompressive. The integrity of the submucosal layer should then be evaluated. Loss of the submucosal layer is seen in gangrenous appendicitis (**Fig. 7**). Presence of Doppler signal is useful in ruling in the diagnosis of appendicitis and increasing confidence; however, absence does not rule it out. Absent Doppler signal can be seen in an inflamed appendix, especially with gangrene (**Fig. 8**).[15,16] The presence of a focal defect in the wall, especially at the tip, should be looked for as an indication of perforation (**Fig. 9**).

The periappendiceal area must then be examined. The degree of secondary thickening of the terminal ileum and cecum should be ascertained. Periappendiceal inflamed fat should be assessed, seen as mass-like, noncompressible, echogenic fat with or without Doppler signal. When inflamed fat is limited to the mesoappendix, it is seen as a triangular-shaped echogenic mass adjacent to the mesenteric side of the appendix (see **Fig. 1D**). When the inflammation extends beyond the mesoappendix, the inflamed fat can become extensive, particularly as the omentum moves in to wall off the process. The presence of a focal

---

Box 2
Signs to rule out appendicitis

Diameter less than 6 mm

Compressible along its entire length

Ovoid in cross section along its entire length

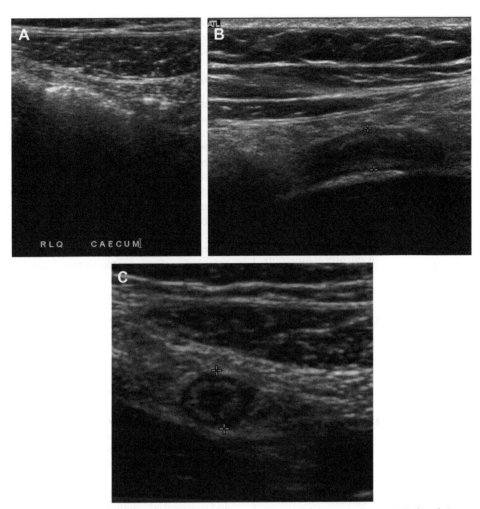

Fig. 6. (*A*) Patient scanned supine—appendix not seen, a potential false-negative on US. (*B, C*) Same patient scanned in the left lateral decubitus position demonstrates an inflamed retrocecal appendix.

collection should be ruled out. A collection less than 4 cm may respond to antibiotics plus or minus image-guided aspiration. A collection greater than 4 cm likely requires percutaneous drainage.

When evaluating patients with appendicitis, two special circumstances can arise. The first is the indeterminate appendix on CT. This is typically an appendix that measures greater than 6 mm in the absence of periappendiceal inflammatory or focal cecal changes. A normal appendix on CT can measure from 2 to 11 mm.[17] One common clinical scenario is a patient sent to CT to rule out renal colic with no renal stone seen and an equivocal appendix. The first option is to administer intravenous contrast to evaluate appendiceal enhancement; however, my preference is evaluate the appendix with a focused US. This allows localization of the point of tenderness and an assessment of the compressibility of the appendix. If normal, the same

appendix that measures greater than 6 mm on CT may compress to less than 6 mm on US (**Fig. 10**).

The second scenario that can arise is the indeterminate appendix on US. Typically this is an appendix that measures 6 mm or 7 mm and is noncompressible. Single wall thickness also is borderline. Doppler signal is absent and tenderness is equivocal. In these cases, it can be difficult to know if the noncompressibility is due to normal content or normal lymphoid tissue. A helpful strategy in these cases, in direct discussion with the referring surgeon, is to follow patients clinically and with a repeat US in 24 hours.

One final point to make regarding appendicitis is in cases when obstruction is not caused by an appendicolith or lymphoid hyperplasia but rather by tumor. A careful evaluation of the base of the appendix on US should avoid the pitfall of missing an obstructing cecal or appendiceal mass. Care should be taken

Table 1
Pitfalls of appendiceal ultrasound

False-Negative Ultrasound	Solution
Unusual position of the appendix	1. Clearly identify the ileocecal valve first 2. Perform transvaginal US in all women if appendix is not seen transabdominally 3. Perform a coronal scan to look for a retrocecal appendix 4. Put the patient in the left lateral decubitus position to look for a retrocecal appendix
Incomplete visualization	1. Ensure demonstration of the blind end

False-Positive Ultrasound	Solution
Mistake a normal appendix for abnormal	1. Short-term follow-up US in discussion with the surgeon for equivocal results on both US and clinical examination 2. When the appendix measures more than 6 mm, also measure the individual wall thickness and evaluate the content 3. Use of Doppler to help rule in appendicitis
Mistake the terminal ileum for the appendix	1. Be rigorous about identifying the ileocecal valve and the blind end of the appendix 2. Terminal ileum is ovoid in cross section, not round, and usually demonstrates peristalsis
Mistake secondary enlargement of the appendix for primary appendicitis • Crohn's disease • Cecal carcinoma or mass • Perforated peptic ulcer disease • Cecal diverticulitis	1. Recognition of the underlying cause 2. Think of an obstructing lesion when the appendix measures greater than 1.5 cm diameter

especially when the diameter of the appendix is more than 15 mm because this has been shown associated with neoplastic obstruction.[18,19]

TERMINAL ILEITIS

Infectious causes of terminal ilieitis, including *Yersinia*, *Campylobacter*, *Salmonella*, and *Shigella*, can cause a clinical presentation identical to that of appendicitis. The role of US in these cases is to diagnose thickening of the terminal ileum and to identify a normal appendix so that surgery is avoided. Bowel wall thickening of the terminal ileum is the predominant feature centered on the inner bowel wall layers. Thickening may also involve the cecum and can extend to involve the entire right colon. The ileocecal valve can be prominent and there is usually mesenteric adenopathy (**Fig. 11**).

INFLAMMATORY BOWEL DISEASE

Inflammatory bowel disease consists of 2 entities, ulcerative colitis (UC) of the large bowel and Crohn's disease. Both can present acutely as a first presentation or with flares and complications of the disease. They are not immune to presenting with a ruptured ovarian cyst, appendicitis, or other bowel pathology and, therefore, a thorough US evaluation must be performed. These patients are often young, requiring many investigations over the course of their disease, and US is ideal to avoid cumulative radiation exposure. Endoscopy is the cornerstone of evaluating inflammatory bowel disease; however, it provides only luminal and mucosal information. US, CT, and MR imaging directly image the bowel wall and the perienteric region. Of these, US is the most cost-effective, the most readily available, and the most suited to repeated examination. It is the only examination at present to offer practical real-time imaging.

CROHN'S DISEASE

Crohn's disease involves the colon alone (30%), the small bowel alone (20%), or both large and small bowel (50%).[20] Although MR imaging and CT enterography and enteroclysis have the highest diagnostic accuracy for the detection of intestinal involvement and extraintestinal complications of Cohn disease, they are not always readily available nor are they well suited to serial examination.[21] US has been shown useful especially in ileal disease (approximately 50% of patients have ileal disease usually over the distal 15–25 cm) but is operator-dependent and requires significant expertise.[22] US is often the initial examination of choice in acute presentations. A meta-analysis of the role of US in diagnosing

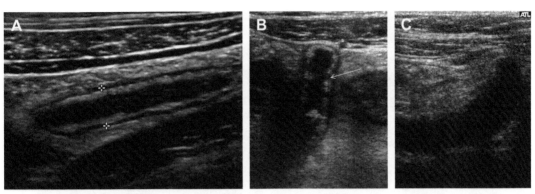

Fig. 7. (A) An abnormal appendix measuring 8 mm in diameter (*between calipers*) with an intact submucosal layer. (B) An abnormal appendix measuring 10 mm in diameter with an irregular submucosal layer (*arrow*). (C) An abnormal appendix measuring 11 mm in diameter with complete loss of the submucosal layer.

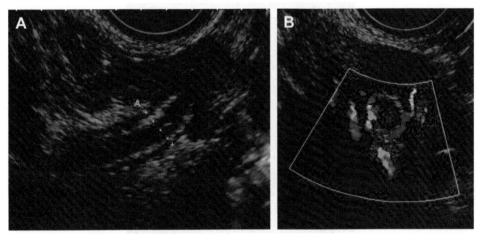

Fig. 8. (A) Abnormal appendix identified only transvaginally, measuring 8 mm. (B) Presence of increased Doppler signal supporting the diagnosis of appendicitis.

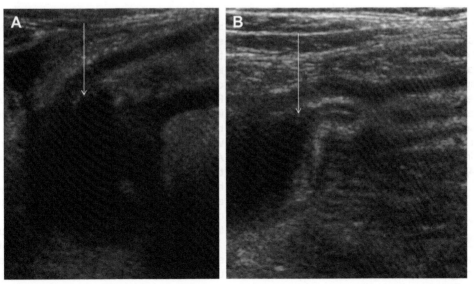

Fig. 9. (A, B) Two separate patients with perforated appendicitis and a focal wall defect at the tip of the appendix (*arrows*).

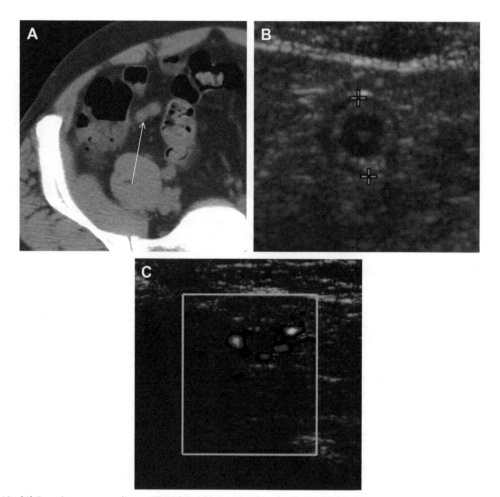

Fig. 10. (*A*) Prominent appendix on CT with no periappendiceal inflammatory change (*arrow*). (*B*) Same appendix on US (*between calipers*), round in cross section, measuring 8 mm, and noncompressible. (*C*) Presence of Doppler signal further confirming appendicitis.

Crohn's disease found a sensitivity of 75% and a specificity of 97% when a bowel wall thickness cutoff of 4 mm was used.[23] US has been shown to be a useful first diagnostic test in patients clinically suspected of having Crohn's disease before proceeding to further more invasive tests.[24–26] It plays a key role in follow-up of patients with known disease, to assess location and extent, and to detect abscesses and strictures. It also can be used in assessment of postoperative recurrence (**Box 4**).[27,28]

Roles 1 and 2: Patients with Acute Right Lower Quadrant Pain or the Initial Evaluation in Suspected Crohn's Disease

The hallmark of Crohn's disease is bowel wall thickening, usually at least moderate, 5 mm to 14 mm.[22] Bowel wall thickening is nonspecific, however, and occurs in other infectious,

inflammatory, and neoplastic conditions. The suspicion of Crohn's disease as a cause is raised, therefore, when the disease is ileocecal in location, is segmental with skip lesions, and in the presence of perienteric findings, such as fistula and abscess. False-negative US occurs when early disease involves the mucosa only, thereby not producing bowel wall thickening. Stratification of the bowel wall is preserved early on in the disease process. As the disease becomes more severe and transmural, the layers become ill defined, finally becoming partially or completely destroyed. In addition the bowel segment is usually stiff and demonstrates reduced or absent peristalsis. Angulation of the bowel may also be appreciated.

Although mucosal disease is the territory of endoscopists, careful evaluation on US can reveal deep ulcers and intramural linear fissures (they may or may not contain gas) in the muscularis mucosa and submucosal layers (**Fig. 12**). Postinflammatory

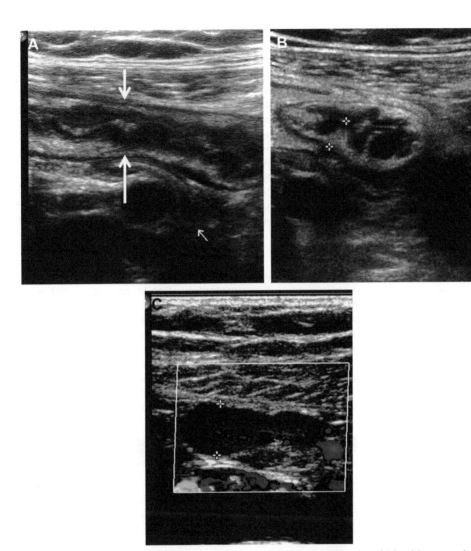

Fig. 11. (*A*) *Yersinia* causing concentric thickening of the terminal ileum (*between thick white arrows*) with preservation of the bowel wall layers. Note the normal appendix (*small white arrow*) posterior to the terminal ileum. (*B*) Wall thickening measuring 5 mm (*between calipers*). (*C*) Mesenteric nodes (*between calipers*).

Box 4
Current roles for ultrasound in Crohn's disease

1. Evaluation of acute patients with right lower quadrant pain

2. Initial evaluation of patients with clinically suspected Crohn's disease

3. Defining anatomic location and extent of disease

4. Detection of complications

5. Follow-up of patients postresection and post–medical therapy

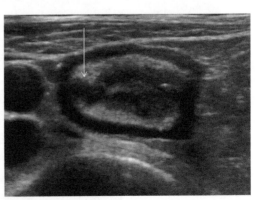

Fig. 12. Initial presentation of Crohn's disease; there is preservation of the bowel wall stratification but the presence of a deep ulcer is seen as a focal disruption of the echogenic submucosal layer (*white arrow*). (*Courtesy of* Dr Josee Sarrazin.)

pseudopolyps are seen as mural nodules, particularly when there is fluid in the bowel lumen.

As with appendicitis, perienteric findings should also be evaluated. The so-called creeping fat of Crohn's disease is seen as mass-like, noncompressible adjacent fat often with linear hypoechoic bands running through it. It is most prominent on the mesenteric side. When chronic it can become heterogeneous or even hypoechoic.[22] It causes loop separation classically described on barium studies but which can also be appreciated on US.

Mesenteric nodes are often seen in Crohn's disease. They usually are hypoechoic, are ovoid in configuration, and measure greater than 5 mm in short axis. They can become conglomerate.

Role 3: Assessing the Location and Extent of Disease

One of the most important factors affecting the accuracy of US in Crohn's disease is the location of disease, with high sensitivity reported for the terminal ileum and left colon and lower sensitivity for the rectum and upper small bowel.[24]

When Crohn's disease is suspected on US, because of its skip nature, a survey of the bowel should be performed as described previously.

Although the ileum is the most common site of disease and one of the easier to localize on US, other sites are discovered if a methodical approach is used. The rectum can be seen with a transvaginal or transperineal scan in women (**Fig. 13**A, B). The duodenum is a blind spot unless specifically looked for.

Role 4: Detection of Complications

Among patients with Crohn's disease, 17% to 82% experience at least one fistula.[27] They are particularly common in the terminal ileum and in the anus. Fistula can occur between the affected segment and adjacent segments of bowel (enteroenteric), to the abdominal wall (enterocutaneous), to the bladder (vesicoenteric), to the vagina, and to the retroperitoneum. They can also blind end in the mesentery. Fistula can occur between the inflamed segment of bowel and an adjacent segment of bowel (enteroenteric), the abdominal wall (enterocutaneous), the bladder (enterovesicle), the vagina or the retroperitoneum. They are often vascular on Doppler and may or may not contain air (**Fig. 14**). Using manual compression can sometimes help move air through the fistula, further confirming its presence on US. US

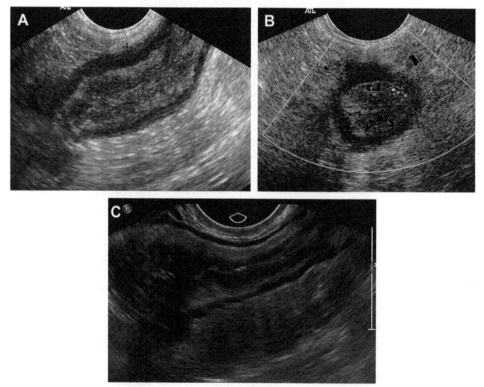

Fig. 13. (*A*) Crohn's disease of the rectum seen transvaginally in the sagittal plane. (*B*) Crohn's disease of the rectum, axial view. (*C*) Crohn's disease of the small bowel—not the terminal ileum—seen only on a transvaginal scan. Note the bowel wall thickening, particularly of the submucosal layer.

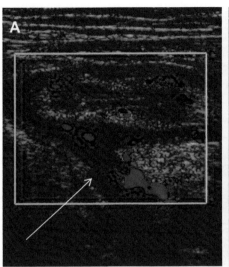 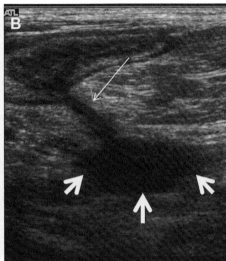

Fig. 14. Two separate patients with fistula secondary to Crohn's disease seen as hypoechoic linear tracts extending beyond the bowel wall into the adjacent tissues. (*A*) A vascular hypoechoic tract (*arrow*). (*B*) A fistula (*long arrow*) leading to a focal abscess (*short arrows*).

is reported in a systematic review to have a 74% sensitivity and a 95% specificity in the diagnosis of Crohn's fistulas.[29]

Abscesses are often the result of a fistula and seen in 12% to 30% of patients.[27] They are commonly found along the mesenteric side, often occurring in the psoas muscle, paracolic gutter, or mesentery of the terminal ileum (see **Fig. 14**B). They are defined as focal collections of fluid often with an irregular wall. They may contain air and debris. By convention they are larger than 2 cm in diameter to differentiate from a blind-ending fistula.[30] US is reported in a systematic review to have an 84% sensitivity and a 93% specificity in the diagnosis of Crohn's abscess.[29]

Strictures occur in up to 21% of people with ileal disease[27] and often require surgery. US has been shown to detect strictures with high accuracy[30–32] as a thickened, stiff loop of affected bowel with a narrow lumen and upstream distended (greater than 3 cm) either fluid-filled or echogenic content-filled bowel.[31] There often is upstream hyperperistalsis. US is reported in a systematic review as having 79% sensitivity and a 92% specificity in the diagnosis of Crohn's stricture.[29]

Role 5: Postsurgical Recurrence

Surgery in the setting of Crohn's disease is used when patients have failed medical management or who have developed complications, such as fistula or stricture. Unfortunately recurrence rates are high. Within 3 years at endoscopy up to 85% to 100% develop recurrence and 34% to 86% if only symptomatic recurrence is considered. US

has been shown to correlate with endoscopy in the detection of postsurgical recurrence (**Fig. 15**).

Disease Activity

Being able to assess disease activity is important in management and prognosis of Crohn's disease. The most widely used method is the clinical Crohn's disease activity index; however, this method has limitations. Lower endoscopy is the method of choice for determining activity in the colon and terminal ileum; however, it is invasive and does not evaluate the remainder of the small bowel. US offers 3 potential techniques for assessing activity. Color Doppler of the superior mesenteric artery[33,34] and Doppler vessel density in the intestine per square centimeter have both been shown to correlate with disease activity but have not entered routine practice.[34–36] Contrast-enhanced US is currently being investigated and may offer increased sensitivity and specificity in terms of assessing disease activity.[35] Gray-scale findings of wall thickness and echo pattern have not proved useful in predicting disease activity. Because the treatment of an inflammatory stricture is medical and a fibrotic stricture surgical, it would be helpful if imaging could distinguish the two. In addition, as newer and more expensive medical therapies are discovered, an objective imaging method to assess disease activity in response to therapy would be useful. This would require serial examinations for which US or contrast-enhanced US are well suited.

Crohn's disease and pregnancy deserve special mention. If disease is in remission at the time of conception, approximately one-third of patients

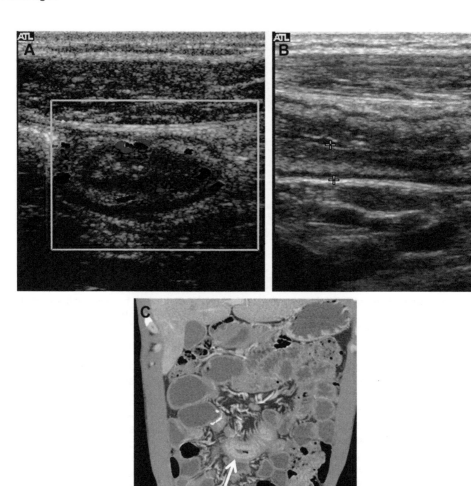

Fig. 15. Recurrence at the neoterminal ileum. (*A*) Cross section of the neoterminal ileum demonstrating bowel wall thickening measuring 7 mm and Doppler signal consistent with inflammation. (*B*) Longitudinal view of the neoterminal ileum; note preservation of bowel wall layers with bowel wall thickening (*between calipers*). (*C*) CT enterogram confirming findings of recurrence at the neoterminal ileum (*arrow*).

will relapse and, therefore, may require imaging. If disease is active during conception, two-thirds of patients will have persistent disease and of this population two-thirds will deteriorate.[36] These numbers, in addition to the safety of US during pregnancy, underscore the necessity for skilled bowel ultrasonographers.

ULCERATIVE COLITIS

UC, in contrast to Crohn's disease, is a condition limited to the colon, occurring continuously from the rectum without skip lesions. Because this disease is colonic and confined to the mucosa, it is particularly well suited to endoscopic

evaluation. US plays much less of a role in UC than it does in Crohn's disease. Although the disease is confined to the mucosa, it can cause thickening of all the layers, especially the submucosa, resulting in bowel wall thickening often up to 5 mm to 10 mm. The muscularis layer, however, is usually normal or only mildly thickened and in general the stratification of the wall is preserved. The deep ulcers of Crohn's disease are not seen in UC. Perienteric findings are typically absent. Pericolonic edema and fluid is uncommon in UC. With chronic disease, there is loss of haustration leading to the lead pipe colon, which is also recognizable on US. Pseudopolyps can be seen as echogenic nodules protruding into the lumen especially when the affected segment contains fluid. Overall it is difficult to reliably distinguish Crohn's colitis from UC and the best predictors are location and presence of perigut disease.[28]

Distinguishing UC from other infectious etiologies is generally not possible on US. Pseudomembranous colitis, however, often causes an accordion sign seen as an exaggeration of the haustra by severe submucosal edema, a sign not generally seen in UC (**Fig. 16**). The thickening is striking, with an effaced lumen, and the outer muscular layer is thin. It is often associated with ascites.[37] In addition the history of recent antibiotic use is helpful.

DIVERTICULITIS

Diverticular disease is a common entity in the Western world; it is estimated that one-third of people over age 40 harbor the disease and that 10% to 25% of people with diverticulosis have at least one episode of acute diverticulitis as a result.[38] As with many conditions discussed in this article, the clinical presentation is nonspecific. Classically patients present with left lower quadrant pain, elevated white count, and fever. Fever and white count, however, are not sensitive, even in the presence of an abscess,[39] underscoring the need for imaging to make a correct diagnosis and to guide management.

There are few studies comparing modalities for diagnosis of diverticulitis and many of them were published before the year 2000; however, US has been shown to have a sensitivity of 85% and a specificity of 84%[40] and CT 91% and 77%, respectively.[31] Because US is often the first test especially in premenopausal women radiologists and ultrasonographers have to be familiar with the findings of diverticulitis on US. A reasonable algorithm in patients with clinically suspected diverticulitis might be to start with US in young

patients in the absence of peritoneal findings. CT could then be performed in the patients who are either inconclusive on US or are found to have large abscesses for consideration of percutaneous drainage.

On US, the diagnosis of diverticulitis is made when there is bowel wall thickening at the site of tenderness measuring more than 4 mm from the inner echogenic interface to the outer edge of the echogenic serosal layer in the presence of an inflamed diverticulum. A diverticulum is a focal outpouching arising from the colonic wall associated with a focal disruption of the bowel layers at its neck. The tic may be hypoechoic, hyperechoic, or hyperechoic with a hypoechoic rim. Content may or may not cause acoustic shadowing (**Fig. 17**). Inflammation is heralded by echogenic noncompressible surrounding fat. Perienteric features should be evaluated, including the presence or absence of extraluminal foci of air, focal fluid collections/abscess, fistula, and adjacent free fluid.

Although diverticulitis is most often a left-sided disease, right-sided diverticulitis is also well recognized. These tics are often congenital true diverticula, meaning that they contain all bowel wall layers. This fact may explain why right-sided diverticulitis is not associated with the complications of abscess, perforation, and fistula seen in left-sided disease. Patients are often younger and clinically can present as identical to appendicitis. It is critical on US to identify the offending tic at the epicenter of inflammation and maximal wall thickening and to document a normal appendix because this disease is treated conservatively. If right-sided diverticulitis is inadvertently sent to

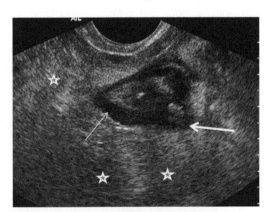

Fig. 17. Transvaginal scan of acute diverticulitis. Note the preferential thickening of the hypoechoic muscular layer rather than the submucosal layer (*thin arrow*). The diverticulum is seen as a focal outpouching projecting beyond the bowel wall, in this case with echogenic nonshadowing content and a hypoechoic rim (*thick arrow*). Surrounding echogenic fat and focal tenderness are consistent with inflammation (*stars*).

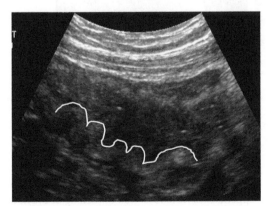

Fig. 16. Accordion sign (tracing) of pseudomembranous colitis, unusual for UC.

the operating room it can result in a right hemicolectomy because the diverticulum is obscured by inflammation and the intraoperative impression is that of a mass rather than diverticulitis (**Fig. 18**).

COLITIS VERSUS TUMOR

GI tumors can present acutely, especially when complicated by perforation. In general, differentiation of acute inflammation, such as diverticulitis from malignancy, can be difficult both clinically and on imaging. It is recommended, therefore, that a first attack of diverticulitis be followed up after the acute presentation with either barium enema or colonoscopy. There are features on US, however, which can be helpful, in particular preservation of the bowel wall layers. Tumor is usually over a shorter segment than inflammation and is bulky with asymmetric involvement. Stratification is lost. Typically perigut features are absent when there is no associated perforation (**Figs. 19** and **20**).[7] If bowel wall layers are lost, with no pericolonic inflammation and in the presence of adjacent nodes, malignancy should be considered. If bowel wall layers are preserved and there is pericolonic inflammatory change, colitis or diverticulitis is more likely.[41]

ISCHEMIA

Multidetector CT is the initial modality of choice in suspected bowel ischemia. On US, ischemia is segmental and generally over a longer length, bowel wall stratification may or may not be preserved, and Doppler signal may be reduced or absent. Absent arterial flow has been associated with a poor outcome.[42] Pericolonic fat changes have been associated with transmural necrosis.[43] Although ischemia is not an indication for US, two situations may arise in which familiarity with US features can aid in arriving at a proper diagnosis.

The first situation is when bowel thickening is seen on CT with no specific features of ischemia and when a differential diagnosis of ischemia versus inflammatory is entertained. Although on US, the degree of bowel wall thickening is not useful, if there is little or absent Doppler signal and no arterial tracings, ischemia is suggested. Readily visible Doppler signal supports inflammation.[44] It is important to ensure that parameters are optimized for sensitivity, including an appropriate filter for low-volume flow, low-velocity scale, wide gate width, and maximal gain (**Fig. 21**).

The second situation is when a patient is referred to US for nonspecific abdominal pain and clinically ischemia has not been suspected. Because the symptoms of ischemia are nonspecific, this is not that unlikely a scenario. In these patients, bowel wall thickening is recognized first, often aided by localizing the point of maximum tenderness with probe pressure. Application of Doppler can then suggest the diagnosis of ischemia, leading to further evaluation with CT (**Fig. 22**).

More recently, contrast US has been investigated in the evaluation of bowel ischemia with positive results but its role in clinical practice is not yet established.[45]

SMALL BOWEL OBSTRUCTION

As with ischemia, multidetector CT is the test of choice in small bowel obstruction. Particularly in

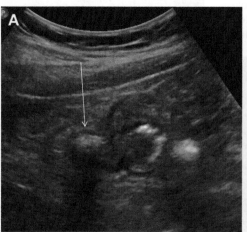 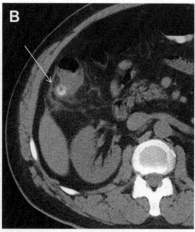

Fig. 18. (A) Young male patient presenting to US to rule out appendicitis. Note focal wall thickening at the neck of a diverticulum (*arrow*) and surrounding echogenic fat. Appendix was seen separately and was normal. (B) Confirmation on CT (*arrow*).

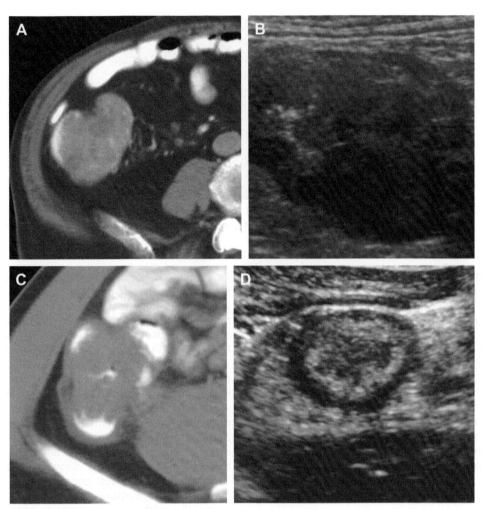

Fig. 19. (*A*) Focal nonspecific thickening on CT involving the right colon in a patient with right lower quadrant pain. (*B*) Same patient on US demonstrating typical features of malignancy, including loss of bowel wall layers and eccentric and bulky short segment thickening. Right colonic adenocarcinoma at scope. (*C*) Separate patient with right lower quadrant pain and nonspecific focal thickening of the right colon on CT. (*D*) Same patient with preservation of bowel wall layers confirming inflammation rather than malignancy.

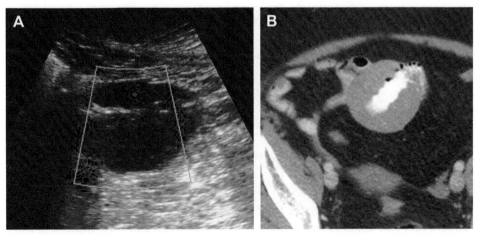

Fig. 20. (*A*) Patient with right lower quadrant pain; short segment of hypoechoic eccentric bowel wall thickening with loss of stratification. (*B*) Same patient at CT. Lymphoma at surgery.

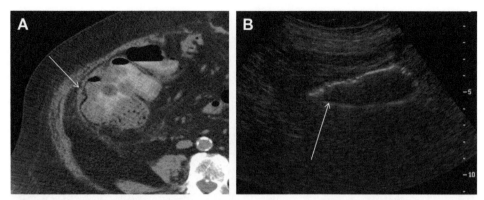

Fig. 21. (*A*) CT scan demonstrated wall thickening of the right colon. Pneumatosis was questioned (*arrow*). Lactate normal. (*B*) US clearly confirmed the presence of pneumatosis (*arrow*) and also showed no Doppler signal (not shown), favoring ischemia over inflammation.

patients who are poor historians or when a language barrier is present, patients can present to US. The inherent fluid-filled nature of obstructed loops makes them well suited to US evaluation. By recognizing and systematically following the dilated loops, the point of obstruction and often the cause is found on US. Obstruction is suspected when the small bowel measures more than 3.0 cm over a length of more than 10 cm and contains increased content. Hyperperistalsis is seen and the valvulae conniventes are obvious. In contrast, ileus usually demonstrates dilated small bowel with reduced peristalsis and the colon may also be dilated.[46]

EPIPLOIC APPENDAGITIS

Epiploic appendages are fatty tags 1 cm to 2 cm thick and 2 cm to 5 cm long that hang from the antimesenteric border of the colon in two longitudinal rows along the tenia. They are most numerous in the sigmoid and cecum.[47] These appendages can twist or the central vein can thrombose, leading to acute pain. Typical patients are younger than those presenting with diverticulitis. Clinically this can mimic the presentation of either diverticulitis or appendicitis. Usually patients can precisely localize the point of their pain, often with 1 finger. Typically associated symptoms, such as diarrhea and nausea, are absent and laboratory findings are normal. Fever is variable. Because the clinical presentation overlaps significantly with epiploic appendagitis and diverticulitis, this becomes a radiologic diagnosis and is an important one to make because treatment is conservative not surgical.

On US, epiploic appendagitis is seen as an ovoid fatty mass adjacent to the colon and immediately beneath the abdominal wall that is tender and noncompressible (**Fig. 23**). The center can

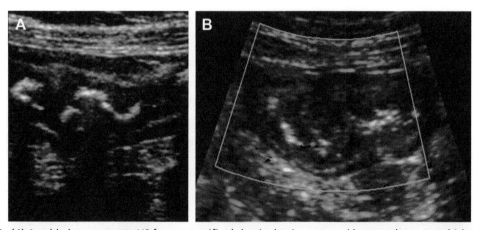

Fig. 22. (*A*) An elderly man sent to US for nonspecific abdominal pain post total knee replacement; thickening of the right colon was associated with tenderness. (*B*) No Doppler signal obtained despite maximizing parameters concerning for ischemia rather than inflammation. CT scan performed. Ischemia confirmed at surgery.

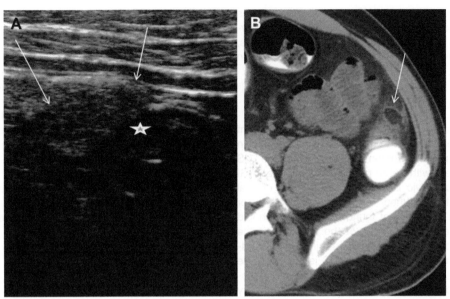

Fig. 23. (*A*) Epiploic appendagitis—a fatty tender mass (*arrows*) adjacent to the left colon. Note the focal eccentric thickening of the outer layer of the left colon (*star*) indicating an adjacent inflammatory process rather than disease of the left colon itself. (*B*) Confirmed on CT (*arrow*).

be hypoechoic secondary to hemorrhage and there is often a thin hypoechoic rim (**Fig. 24**). There may be associated focal thickening of the adjacent colonic wall but the colonic wall should not be circumferentially thickened. The mass moves with the colon on respiration and can often also be fixed to the adjacent peritoneum. Doppler signal is typically absent (in contrast to diverticulitis).[47] On the right, a normal appendix must be documented, and on the left, a careful

search should be made for an underlying inflamed diverticulum.

OMENTAL INFARCTION

Omental infarction is far less common than epiploic appendagitis. It usually occurs on the right side and can present as similar to appendicitis. As with epiploic appendagitis, management is conservative. The normal appendix must be

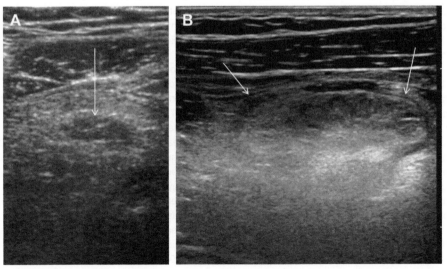

Fig. 24. (*A*) Epiploic appendagitis on US demonstrating a hypoechoic center (*arrow*). (*B*) Another patient with epiploic appendagitis demonstrating a fatty mass with a hypoechoic rim (*arrows*). (*Courtesy of* Dr Laurent Milot.)

demonstrated. Omental infarction also presents as a hyperechoic noncompressible fatty mass; however, it is usually larger than epiploic appendagitis. It is located anterior to the right colon and is often adherent to the peritoneum.[48,49]

SUMMARY

In summary, US of the bowel requires significant expertise but is extremely useful, especially in premenopausal women presenting to the US department with pelvic pain. Gynecologic and GI causes of pelvic pain can cause similar clinical presentations. When a gynecologic cause for a patient's pain is not found, the GI tract should be evaluated. Knowledge of the anatomy of the bowel wall and the GI tract is required. A methodical approach must be used. US is known to be accurate in the diagnosis of appendicitis, diverticulitis, and inflammatory bowel disease. Familiarity with the features of small bowel obstruction and intestinal ischemia prevent misdiagnosis and allow proper use of further imaging.

REFERENCES

1. Andreotti RF, Lee SI, DeJesus Allison SO, et al. ACR appropriateness criteria: acute pelvic pain in the reproductive age group. Ultrasound Q 2011;27: 205–10.
2. Cammarota T, Sarno A, Robotti D, et al. US evaluation of patients affected by IBD: how to do it, methods and findings. Eur J Radiol 2009;69:429–37.
3. Puylaert JB. Acute appendicitis: US evaluation using graded compression. Radiology 1986;158:355–60.
4. Lee JH, Jeong YK, Hwang JC, et al. Graded compression sonography with adjuvant use of a posterior manual compression technique in the sonographic diagnosis of acute appendicitis. Am J Roentgenol 2002;178:863–8.
5. Maconi G, Radice E, Bareggi E, et al. Hydrosonography of the gastrointestinal tract. Am J Roentgenol 2009;193:700–8.
6. Pallotta N, Vincoli G, Montesani C, et al. Small intestine contrast ultrasonography (SICUS) for the detection of small bowel complications in Crohn's disease: a prospective comparative study versus intraoperative findings. Inflamm Bowel Dis 2011. [Epub ahead of print].
7. Truong M, Atri M, Bret PM, et al. Sonographic appearance of benign and malignant conditions of the colon. Am J Roentgenol 1998;170:1451–5.
8. Frisoli JK, Desser TS, Jeffrey RB. Thickened submucosal layer. Am J Roentgenol 2000;175:1595–9.
9. Addiss DG, Shaffer N, Fowler BS, et al. The epidemiology of appendicitis and appendectomy in the United States. Am J Epidemiol 1990;132:910–25.
10. Bendeck SE, Nino-Murcia M, Berry GJ, et al. Imaging for suspected appendicitis: negative appendectomy and perforation rates1. Radiology 2002;225:131–6.
11. van Randen A, Bipat S, Zwinderman AH, et al. Acute appendicitis: meta-analysis of diagnostic performance of ct and graded compression US related to prevalence of disease1. Radiology 2008;249:97–106.
12. Rettenbacher T, Hollerweger A, Macheiner P, et al. Outer diameter of the vermiform appendix as a sign of acute appendicitis: evaluation at US1. Radiology 2001;218:757–62.
13. Rettenbacher T, Hollerweger A, Macheiner P, et al. Ovoid shape of the vermiform appendix: a criterion to exclude acute appendicitisâ€"evaluation with US1. Radiology 2003;226:95–100.
14. Rioux M. Sonographic detection of the normal and abnormal appendix. Am J Roentgenol 1992;158: 773–8.
15. Chan L, Shin LK, Pai RK, et al. Pathologic continuum of acute appendicitis: sonographic findings and clinical management implications. Ultrasound Q 2011;27:71–9.
16. Quillin SP, Siegel MJ. Appendicitis: efficacy of color Doppler sonography. Radiology 1994;191:557–60.
17. Benjaminov O, Atri M, Hamilton P, et al. Frequency of visualization and thickness of normal appendix at nonenhanced helical CT1. Radiology 2002;225: 400–6.
18. Lien WC, Huang SP, Chi CL, et al. Appendiceal outer diameter as an indicator for differentiating appendiceal mucocele from appendicitis. Am J Emerg Med 2006;24:801–5.
19. Pickhardt PJ, Levy AD, Rohrmann CA, et al. Primary neoplasms of the appendix manifesting as acute appendicitis: CT findings with pathologic comparison1. Radiology 2002;224:775–81.
20. Valette PJ, Rioux MR, Pilleul FP, et al. Ultrasonography of chronic inflammatory bowel diseases. Eur Radiol 2001;11:1859–66.
21. Van Assche G, Dignass A, Panes J, et al. The second European evidence-based consensus on the diagnosis and management of Crohn's disease: definitions and diagnosis. J Crohns Colitis 2010;4: 7–27.
22. Sarrazin J, Wilson SR. Manifestations of Crohn disease at US. Radiographics 1996;16:499–520.
23. Fraquelli M, Colli A, Casazza G, et al. Role of US in detection of crohn disease: meta-analysis1. Radiology 2005;236:95–101.
24. Parente F, Greco S, Molteni M, et al. Role of early ultrasound in detecting inflammatory intestinal disorders and identifying their anatomical location within the bowel. Aliment Pharmacol Ther 2003;18: 1009–16.
25. Solvig J, Ekberg O, Lindgren S, et al. Ultrasound examination of the small bowel: comparison with

enteroclysis in patients with Crohn disease. Abdom Imaging 1995;20:323–6.

26. Astegiano M, Bresso F, Cammarota T, et al. Abdominal pain and bowel dysfunction: diagnostic role of intestinal ultrasound. Eur J Gastroenterol Hepatol 2001;13:927–31.

27. Maconi G, Radice E, Greco S, et al. Bowel ultrasound in Crohn's disease. Best Pract Res Clin Gastroenterol 2006;20:93–112.

28. Onali S, Calabrese E, Petruzziello C, et al. Endoscopic vs ultrasonographic findings related to Crohn's disease recurrence: a prospective longitudinal study at 3 years. J Crohns Colitis 2010;4:319–28.

29. Panés J, Bouzas R, Chaparro M, et al. Systematic review: the use of ultrasonography, computed tomography and magnetic resonance imaging for the diagnosis, assessment of activity and abdominal complications of Crohn's disease. Aliment Pharmacol Ther 2011;34:125–45.

30. Gasche C, Moser G, Turetschek K, et al. Transabdominal bowel sonography for the detection of intestinal complications in Crohn's disease. Gut 1999;44:112–7.

31. Parente F, Maconi G, Bollani S, et al. Bowel ultrasound in assessment of Crohn's disease and detection of related small bowel strictures: a prospective comparative study versus x ray and intraoperative findings. Gut 2002;50:490–5.

32. Maconi G, Bollani S, Bianchi Porro G. Ultrasonographic detection of intestinal complications in Crohn's disease. Dig Dis Sci 1996;41:1643–8.

33. Miao YM, Koh DM, Amin Z, et al. Ultrasound and magnetic resonance imaging assessment of active bowel segments in Crohn's disease. Clin Radiol 2002;57:913–8.

34. Karoui S, Nouira K, Serghini M, et al. Assessment of activity of Crohn's disease by Doppler sonography of superior mesenteric artery flow. J Crohns Colitis 2010;4:334–40.

35. Migaleddu V, Scanu AM, Quaia E, et al. Contrast-enhanced ultrasonographic evaluation of inflammatory activity in Crohn's disease. Gastroenterology 2009;137:43–52.

36. Van Assche G, Dignass A, Reinisch W, et al. The second European evidence-based Consensus on the diagnosis and management of Crohn's disease: special situations. J Crohns Colitis 2010;4:63–101.

37. Downey DB, Wilson SR. Pseudomembranous colitis: sonographic features. Radiology 1991;180:61–4.

38. Liljegren G, Chabok A, Wickbom M, et al. Acute colonic diverticulitis: a systematic review of diagnostic accuracy. Colorectal Dis 2007;9:480–8.

39. Bruel JM. Acute colonic diverticulitis: CT or ultrasound? Eur Radiol 2003;13:2557–9.

40. Pradel JA, Adell JF, Taourel P, et al. Acute colonic diverticulitis: prospective comparative evaluation with US and CT. Radiology 1997;205:503–12.

41. Chintapalli KN, Chopra S, Ghiatas AA, et al. Diverticulitis versus colon cancer: differentiation with helical CT findings. Radiology 1999;210:429–35.

42. Danse EM, Van Beers BE, Jamart J, et al. Prognosis of ischemic colitis. Am J Roentgenol 2000;175:1151–4.

43. Ripolles T, Simo L, Martinez-Perez M, et al. Sonographic findings in ischemic colitis in 58 patients. Am J Roentgenol 2005;184:777–85.

44. Teefey SA, Roarke MC, Brink JA, et al. Bowel wall thickening: differentiation of inflammation from ischemia with color Doppler and duplex US. Radiology 1996;198:547–51.

45. Hata J, Kamada T, Haruma K, et al. Evaluation of bowel ischemia with contrast-enhanced US: initial experience1. Radiology 2005;236:712–5.

46. Schmutz GR, Benko A, Fournier L, et al. Small bowel obstruction: role and contribution of sonography. Eur Radiol 1997;7:1054–8.

47. Almeida AT, Melão L, Viamonte B, et al. Epiploic appendagitis: an entity frequently unknown to clinicians: diagnostic imaging, pitfalls, and look-alikes. Am J Roentgenol 2009;193:1243–51.

48. Puylaert JB. Right-sided segmental infarction of the omentum: clinical, US, and CT findings. Radiology 1992;185:169–72.

49. McClure MJ, Khalili K, Sarrazin J, et al. Radiological features of epiploic appendagitis and segmental omental infarction. Clin Radiol 2001;56:819–27.

Index

Note: Page numbers of article titles are in **boldface** type.

Ultrasound Clin 7 (2012) 155–160
doi:10.1016/S1556-858X(11)00158-7

Moving?

Make sure your subscription moves with you!

To notify us of your new address, find your **Clinics Account Number** (located on your mailing label above your name), and contact customer service at:

Email: journalscustomerservice-usa@elsevier.com

800-654-2452 (subscribers in the U.S. & Canada)
314-447-8871 (subscribers outside of the U.S. & Canada)

Fax number: 314-447-8029

Elsevier Health Sciences Division
Subscription Customer Service
3251 Riverport Lane
Maryland Heights, MO 63043

*To ensure uninterrupted delivery of your subscription, please notify us at least 4 weeks in advance of move.

ELSEVIER

Printed and bound by CPI Group (UK) Ltd, Croydon, CR0 4YY

03/10/2024

01040358-0009